MR. SAL'S EXCELLENT GUIDE
to Better Grooming, Etiquette, and the Man Rules

Mr. Sal Cipolla

*Mr. Sal's Excellent Guide
to Better Grooming, Etiquette, and the Man Rules*

©2020. Sal Cipolla. All rights reserved.

No part of this book may be reproduced or transmitted in any form or by any means, electronic or mechanical, including photocopying, recording, or by an information storage and retrieval system without written permission of the publisher.

ISBN: 978-1-948261-37-1
LOCC 2020909807

Cover Design & Interior Layout: Christa Mella

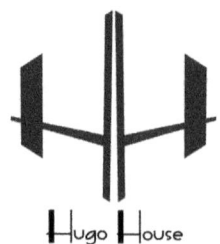

Hugo House Publishers, Ltd.
Austin, TX • Englewood, CO
www.HugoHousePublishers.com

For Paula Sinnard,
Who was the inspiration and continues to inspire.

Table of Contents

Introduction	7
The List	11
Bathing and Skincare	13
Mirror, Mirror	27
Apparel	33
Etiquette	51
The Man Rules	71
The Grasshopper and the Ant	85
Acknowledgements	91
About the Author	93

INTRODUCTION

A few years back, during my many pursuits of different jobs, professions, and adventures, had the occasion to work side by side with a fellow whom I'll call Bryan. In our capacity as security guards for a major university in New York City, Bryan and I would greet students and faculty alike, walk the halls of learning, check all the doors and passages, and generally sit on our bums reading the newspaper. Such is the menial life of a security guard.

Bryan had a special penchant for the ladies. His constant obsequious behavior towards the fairer sex would elicit a response ranging from hidden repulsion to an uncomfortable, "thank you," followed by a quick getaway. In Bryan's defense, he was a stout young male with a strong jaw, straight nose, lively blue eyes, and an affable demeanor. Notwithstanding his somewhat inappropriate behavior, Bryan was a fairly pleasant fellow. So what was the problem? One day while "all quiet on the western front" Bryan's conversation turned from how bad the Mets were playing to something of a personal nature.

"Hey Sal, let me ask you something...you're a man of the world, been around the block a few times, seen some things...why is it I can't seem to get a date? I mean I think I'm a good looking guy?"

I nodded in agreement.

"So what's the problem?" he asked. "Be straight with me."

I turned around on my swivel chair, and leaned in face to face. "You want the truth?" I asked?

He nodded in the affirmative.

And there it was, that strange awkward, cumbersome moment we've all experienced when someone asks you to "give it to them straight." I took a deep breath.

"Bryan," I said, "have you ever looked at yourself in the mirror, I mean really taken a good look at yourself?"

"Yea...what of it?"

"Well, besides the fact it looks like you've entered your eyebrows in an Andy Rooney look-a-like contest, you have these really long hairs coming out of your nose! It's disgusting!"

To wit he replied, "So what should I do about them?"

"What are you, a schmuck? Cut them!"

And then, dear reader, with that perpetual incredulousness that many unkempt, slovenly men have answered in the past he said, "But won't they grow back thicker?"

To wit I proclaimed, "Well, then you cut them again. You shave every day, right?"

The lesson of this small tale is simple: Accentuate the positive, eliminate the negative. If you have a unibrow, shave it in the middle. I promise you, after a few times, it won't grow back. (These and other tips will be covered in the section on hair.)

The number one rule in good grooming is this: Vanity is good! Why do you think most women look good all the time? Because they make it their business to do so. They carry the tools of grooming with them. I must confess that most of the grooming tips in this book come from my years of social intercourse with women. Always conscious of style, fashion trends, new innovations in hair products and cosmetics, women are light-years ahead of the average Joe.

Mind you I'm not suggesting we start carrying handbags, after all we're still men, but not having to primp as much as women, gives us a considerable advantage. The mores of men's fashion and grooming trends tend to stay stable much longer than the ever-fluctuating cacophony of women's products and accessories. In other words, a well-made tailored suit, a few solid pairs of well-crafted footwear, a small array of fitted dress shirts with matching ties, and some casual wear, if properly cared for, should stay in style for a considerable amount of time. Hang onto your clothes because sooner or later they may come back in fashion. Remember bell bottoms and leisure suits...who knows? As the words to the song go, "The girls go crazy for a sharp dressed man." Men do too, (depending on your preference).

The other side of being a well-groomed and well-rounded male has to do with etiquette. The Oxford English Dictionary defines etiquette as: "the customary code of polite behavior in society…."or among "members of a certain professions…" In this fast paced world of instant news and social information, it seems to me that some of the common courtesies of yesteryear have flown out the window. An article that I read in *Psychology Today*, a few years back, stated that, as they phrased it, "a rash of rudeness" has permeated our society. I totally concur. Acts of chivalrous kindness may seem antiquated, and out of date to some, but as men, I believe it's up to us to keep the torch aflame.

Over the years I have witnessed many things, good and bad. But of late it seems to me that society's lack of empathy and compassion for our fellow beings is at an all-time high. Call me a pessimist if you like, but in truth we live inside our own life's experiences and form our opinions from how we view the world around us.

Recently, while dining alfresco at a local bistro, a young lady sitting a few tables over from me and my guest, stumbled and fell as she tried to maneuver her way up to leave. Some young lads standing behind her drinking beer did nothing but gawk at her misfortune. No one came to her rescue, not even the woman sitting at the next table. She was standing, as I and the waiter made our way towards her, and politely asked if she was alright. The young lady nodded in the affirmative, but the incredulity in her expression was obvious; not one gentleman in the bunch.

The simple act of opening a door for someone, offering your seat on a crowded train, or helping someone carry their groceries seems to have diminished over my lifetime. And these acts of kindness have been replaced with more insidious incivilities such as texting while someone is speaking to you, speaking out loud on your cell phone with no consideration for those around you, and taking all the time in the world when it's your turn at the bank or supermarket with no concern for others. You get the picture. We've become a society of "Me." The rule here is simple: always be a gentleman in all walks of life. Women will notice and appreciate your efforts.

So here dear readers, is Mr. Sal's little book of grooming tips and other suggestions. Hopefully, you will find it informative, instructive, and fun on your journey to becoming a dashing, stylish, and well-groomed man.

1

The List

Before we begin your journey to becoming that irresistible, dashing Beau Brummell* that women want to be around and men envy, you're going to need a few things. A grooming grocery list if you will. Some of these items you might already have, some you might not need right away, and some you might add on your own. Don't be afraid to experiment. Some are inexpensive, some are costly, but consider the fact that the average woman spends about $800 a year on beauty supplies. I promise you it won't cost that much to look good!

1. A magnifying mirror is essential for all aspects of skincare and hair grooming. (This can be purchased at any good department store. I have one that lights up)

2. A small toiletry or travel case. Makes sense to keep these items in the same place and you'll always be ready for a trip.

3. A good hair brush and comb.

4. A nail clipper kit: nail and toenail clipper, nail file, cuticle stick, and a sturdy emery board.

5. Tweezers and small barber scissors.

6. Firming and anti-wrinkle cream. (You could go with name brand, but most generic products work just as well and are not as costly.)

7. Astringent; I use 70% rubbing alcohol.

8. Hemorrhoid ointment. (I'll explain later)

9. A facial cleansing buff/plastic loofah/back brush/hand and fingernail brush.

10. Talcum or baby powder.

11. Paper towels.

12. Electric trimmer/razor.

13. Lint brush, coat brush.

14. Shoe brush/shoe horn.

15. A good cologne of your choosing.

This list, like just about everything in life, is not etched in stone. I've probably left out a few essentials, but this should suffice to get you started.

* see chapter on apparel

2

Bathing & Skincare

The Shower vs. the Bath.
Who invented the shower? The answer is simple, nature. Indigenous peoples in mostly warm climates would bathe under a natural waterfall and rinse themselves in the waters below. Even the ancient Greeks and Romans would occasionally pump water through a small aqueduct, and cleanse themselves in this manner. But for most of recorded history and almost all of European times, people took baths. For one very important reason; the ability to heat the water. As a matter of fact, the city of Bath in England, which was founded by the Romans in about 60 B.C.E., is named Bath for its strategic location to a hot spring. The Romans who loved to bathe, built bathhouses and spas, rubbed their bodies with scented oils, took steam baths, massages, and spoke of continual world domination. They were a fun bunch.

During medieval times, bathing more than one a week was quite a chore even for the aristocracy. Vast amounts of water had to be heated, tubs filled and drained, and it wasn't uncommon for entire families to bathe together. In the seventeenth and eighteenth centuries most Europeans smelled pretty foul. Perfume was used to mask the odors. Heads were shaved to rid oneself of lice, and replaced with wigs. And through it all heavy woolen clothing and elaborate brocade carried the sweat and smells of the city. (Must have been delightful.)

Dental hygiene was almost nonexistent as most rubbed their teeth with a useless cloth. If that wasn't enough, some believed bathing was detrimental to your health. The medical thinking of the day was that airborne germs (miasmas) entered your body through your skin pores and caused a myriad of diseases. Since bathing in hot water opens your pores, you were most susceptible at this point, and many a Duke and Countess were known to bathe in their undergarments.

America wasn't much better as the bath was the predominant source of cleansing oneself, especially in the colder northern climates. The standing bath, or sponge bath as it became known, was the daily ritual if you were lucky. I read somewhere that the first showers in America made their debut in New Orleans. Founded by the French, these primitive showers were referred to as "Douche Baths." America certainly didn't invent the shower, but we most assuredly made it an art form. Using less water than a bath, and considerably less time, it became a perfect fit for our get-up and go mindset.

I was surprised to find, during the year I spent in England, that the house I lived in did not have a shower, and that many Europeans prefer baths to this day.

Most of us know there are three kinds of showers. The first we'll call the quickie, or the military shower, not to be confused with the "Navy Shower," which involves turning the water on and off. This basically is the three minute shower. My father told me when he was in the Air Force that this was common practice. A minute to wet, a minute to scrub, and a minute to rinse. (Having a G.I. haircut obviously makes this process much easier.) Anyone reading this has already taken a thousand quickie showers to avoid being late for work, or an appointment, so this is not news. The second kind is your everyday, take-a- little bit more time to soak yourself and wash behind your ears, shower. This method will more than suffice. So let's move on.

The third kind of shower I refer to as The Leisure Shower. This is when you have the time to relax and wash yourself thoroughly and truly enjoy the therapeutic benefits of a warm shower.

How to Shower Properly.

1. Before you turn on the water, stand in the tub or shower area, and with your back brush or a body brush, gently scrub your skin. This removes dead skin cells. If you can afford to, face the shower head towards the wall turn the water full force on extreme hot. Let the steam fill the shower area, and for a few minutes let the steam immerse your body.

2. You want the water temperature to be warm, not hot. Wet yourself all over, and begin washing from the top down.

3. Wash your hair first. Using gravity while showering makes sense. I suggest a basic shampoo with not a lot of fragrance or additives. Follow the instructions on the product label and use an equally basic conditioner. (I am of the belief that it is not necessary to wash your hair everyday. Washing it every other day, or every three days, saves the natural oils produced by your scalp.)

4. Before you wash your face, make sure your soap is free from fragrance and deodorants. Use a basic soap. (I use Ivory soap and have all my life.) Take your face cleansing buff, soap it up, and in circular motions vigorously scrub your face. Make sure you scrub behind your ears, the back and front of your neck, and along the hairline. Rinse.

5. Taking your hand brush, scrub your hands and fingernails.

6. Now with your body loofah, continue with the rest of your body, working your way down to your feet.

7. With back brush in hand, wash your back vigorously. Rinse.

8. There are more germs on your feet than any other part of your body. Having a separate brush for your feet makes sense, but if not, use your back brush and really scrub your feet. Get in between the toes, the bottoms, and the heels. Rinse.

9. Before you exit the shower, adjust the water temperature to as cool as you can stand it, and rinse yourself again. This will close your skin pores and refresh you.

10. With a clean towel, gently pat yourself dry.

The Standing Bath or Sponge Bath

Let's be honest. If you live in a part of the world where winter rears its ugly head, and the cold winds blow, taking a shower at times can be an uncomfortable experience. I was born and raised in New York City and remember those single digit days of boiling water on the stove just to generate some heat in my one room flat. The idea of jumping out of bed when it was eight degrees outside and dealing with the fluctuating water temperature of an old apartment building is not my fondest memory. To put it bluntly—I hate the cold! Many a day I resorted to bathing myself as quickly and expediently as possible. This procedure is also good if you really need to fly.

1. Wash your face in the sink first.

2. Undress and squat in the tub, turning on the bath faucet.

3. Adjust the temperature to your liking.

4. With a bath sponge or loofah, wash your underarms, your privates, your feet, and as much of your body you deem necessary.

5. Rinse with the sponge and you're done.

6. Dry yourself. Apply some talcum or baby powder, and you're good to go.

Dry Cleaning Your Body

This is something I do when I need to freshen up.

First, wash your face. Pour some 70 percent alcohol on a paper towel and wipe your face, underarms, and as much of your body as you like. Apply some talcum powder and a dab of cologne.

Nails

A few interesting facts about your nails:

1. Nails and hair are made up of the same protein, keratin. So a diet rich in fruits, veggies, protein, and minerals is great for both.

2. Men's nails grow faster than women's. And nails in general grow faster in warm weather.

3. Your nails, according to medical research, are a window to other bodily conditions; any blatant discoloration or unusual discomfort should be checked out. That goes for your toenails as well.

4. As you age, so do your nails. Seniors tend to have more health problems in this area. Keeping nails healthy all your life makes sense.

5. Biting your nails is called onychophagia. Most of us suffer from this when we're young, and tend to grow out of this insidious habit by the time we're adults. So the next time you see some young lad biting his nails say, "Stop being an onychophagist!" At the very least, he'll stop biting long enough to look up the word.

6. Your cuticles are there for a reason. They keep moisture and germs out, and for this reason it is advisable not to cut your cuticles.

7. Stress is bad for your nails. (As we now know, stress is bad for everything.)

How to Give Yourself a Manicure

It seems odd to me that the one hand treatment women do the most, and men do the least, should be called a "MAN-i-cure." The etymology of the word manus simply means "Hand," so take out your nail kit and let's get started.

1. On a flat surface, place a hand towel or placemat. The darker in color the better.

2. With a small nail file, remove all the dead skin and dirt under the nail by gently running the edge of the file under each nail.

3. Clip your nails to a desired length.

4. With the shaping side of the nail file, file each finger following the natural curve of the tip of your finger.

5. Once that's done, take your emery board and smooth each finger rubbing away any dead skin or imperfections.

6. Soak your fingers in warm to moderately hot water for a few minutes.

7. Using the cuticle stick, push the cuticle back starting from the top of the nail working each finger individually. If you have any hanging skin, or cuticle debris, use a cuticle cutter.

8. Rub some hand lotion or nail cream on each nail.

9. If you like, apply a small amount of satin finish clear nail polish.

The Man's Pedicure

There's a lot more to getting a professional pedicure than just clipping your toenails. And if you ever have the chance, or the inclination, I suggest you have one done. But for now, I'll give you the short version of what I call The Man Pedicure:

I usually do this procedure before I take a shower:

1. Find a place where you can put your feet up and sit at the same time. A small stool I have at home seems to work best for me.

2. With your nail file once again, remove all dirt and dead skin from under your toenails.

3. With the toenail clipper, cut each nail as straight across as you can.

4. With the rough side of your emery board or footboard, file each individual nail, covering as much of the surface as you can.

5. With a pumice stone, rub away as much dead, rough skin as possible, Example: the heel, arch, under the toes, and etc.

6. Shower, or wash your feet.

7. With the cuticle stick, push the cuticle back as far as it will go.

8. Apply your lotion or nail cream to each toe.

9. If you have any unwanted hairs on your toes or feet , with a disposable razor, gently shave them off. Your feet will look better and smell better. Another good idea is to occasionally soak your feet in Epsom salts. This will help kill off fungus and germs, and your feet will thank you for it.

Skincare

Do you know what the largest organ of the human body is? You guessed it, your skin. Very few people have perfect skin for a myriad of reasons: bad diet, acne scars, genetics, eczema, smoking, drinking, unsightly moles and abrasions, not washing or exfoliating enough, or working in a job with chemicals or detergents. Most of these problems can be solved by taking care of your skin.

There's a reason why every woman you've ever known rubs lotions and creams on her body after a shower, or before going to sleep. First thing you need to know is what type of skin you have. Is your skin oily, or somewhere in between? Or, are you one of the few who has a perfect pH balance? PH balance, which stands for Potential Hydrogen or Power Hydrogen, is the measure of how much acidity versus alkaline is in any given substance. Your skin has a pH balance, and that pH balance has a number. The perfect pH number is 7, and anything above or below means your skin is either too acidic or too alkaline.

Now this is not a health book, nor do I profess to have anything more than a mild understanding of skin chemistry, but I know my own body. I've always had skin that was too acidic which made it more oily. As a youth, I suffered from pimples, pustular eruptions, blemishes, and the usual adolescent skin maladies. Part of the reason was I didn't wash my face properly, and not often enough. Putting any type of lotion or salve on my face at that time would mean disaster. As I aged, my skin has lost much of its acidic properties and became easier to deal with. So first, know your own skin. Second, and I can't stress this enough: If you want clear skin, wash and exfoliate your face daily if possible.

Washing Your Face

1. Wash your face every morning, but more importantly, every night before you retire.

A good idea is to have two cleansing buffs. Keep one in the shower and the other accessible to the sink area.

2. If you have bad skin, allow me to suggest a technique I've used in the past. It will take some time, and a little effort, but it's well worth it. The only other item you will need to do this, besides your soap and cleansing buff, is apple cider vinegar.

   a. Making sure your sink is clean, fill it up with water as hot as you can stand it.

   b. Soap up your cleansing buff and scrub your face.

   c. With the same water, rinse your face 30 times.

   d. Drain the sink, wash it out, and fill it again as hot as you can stand it.

   e. Pour a substantial amount of the apple cider vinegar into the water.

   f. Rinse your face 15 times with the vinegar water. Drain the sink.

   g. With cold running water, gently splash your face 3 or 4 times.

h. With a clean towel, gently pat your face dry.

I promise you if you do this daily, within a few weeks, you will see a noticeable difference in the texture and radiance of your skin.

Tighten Up Your Face

There are many products made for facial skin care. Most of them are produced for women. If you go into any large drugstore chain, there are more than a few aisles devoted specifically to women's cosmetics and beauty aids. The men's department is usually in the back of the store, takes up a tenth of the aisle, and consists of nothing more than a few types of hair treatments, dyes, shaving cream, some deodorants, and the ever present bottle of Old Spice. (You'd think they would at least put the condoms in this area, but they always seem to be somewhere else.)

There's a reason for this sporadic product displacement. Men don't spend anywhere near the amount of money women do on these sorts of products. If you wish to buy some of the products I'm suggesting you'll have to play in their ballpark. I understand that this may be a bit uncomfortable, and even I get self-conscience at times, walking around in the cosmetic aisle looking for eye cream or facial masque. But you'd be astonished how helpful the women working at these establishments are when waiting on a man. (Maybe they're trying to tell us something?)

Facial Masque

There are many different types of facial masque, some are used for deep cleaning, and others to hydrate the skin, but most of these products help tighten the skin, remove blackheads, and refine your pores. If you have oily skin, you want to buy one that is clay based. If your skin is dry a hydrating masque is preferred. The best way to apply a face masque is before you shower.

Avocado Masque: Pit an avocado, and with a blender or food processor, create a paste, and apply it to your face. It contains vitamin E, and has a soothing and softening effect.

Microdermabrasion: What exactly is microdermabrasion? Basically, it removes a fine layer of skin known as the "Stratum Corneum," and has been touted as an instant facelift. You could spend the money and have this done by an esthetician, but if you go online, you'll find an array of do-it-yourself products ranging in price from $100 – $300. What I suggest is the Olay Microdermabrasion Kit. It's relatively inexpensive and it does a great job. However, this is not to be done every day. And the kit holds about three applications. This is another product that's best used before you shower.

Baking Soda: You might also want to try this homegrown method of exfoliating your skin. Take some baking soda mix it with a little warm water, making a viscous mud, and with your facial buff, using circular motions, gently wash your face. You can do this natural procedure a few times a week as the fine granules will not scrape or damage your skin. You can also do this on any part of your body where you suffer from dry skin. Rinse with warm water.

To Be or Not to Be?

Here's a little trick I learned from years of being an actor. Remember the eighth item on **The List** Hemorrhoid ointment? Well, squeeze out a small amount of the ointment and a small amount of your anti-wrinkle firming cream. Mix together in the palm of your hand and apply some of the mixture under your eyes, crow's feet, and laugh lines; rub the remainder on your neck. Wipe off the excess when necessary. This will tighten your skin and give you an instant eye lift. Best time to do this is an hour or so before you go out on the town. I know this seems a little strange, but it works.

Run for Cover

I broach the subject of men's cosmetics with trepidation. I know some of you will read this and say, "that's where I draw the line Mr. Sal, I'm not gonna start wearing makeup." But from my years of being in show-biz, I've learned the benefits of a little cover. We all have imperfections of our skin, and this small step will help in masking those flaws. If applied sparingly, no one will ever notice. I know purchasing this product is as uncomfortable as buying condoms in the days when you had to ask the pharmacist. (Oy! Was that a drag.)

First step is finding a shade that matches your complexion. A liquid-based foundation is best. Walk boldly into the cosmetic aisle, find a brand you think might work, and when the nice young lady asks if you need any help, lie. "My girlfriend asked me to get her some cover makeup, I know it's this brand, but I don't know what shade?"

To wit she'll inquire, "Well what's her complexion like?"

You say, "Like mine I guess." She will pick something out that suits you, probably know you're lying, and ask you if you need any makeup wedges, (which you do), but if the product is right for you, you'll never have to ask again.

Or, you could punch yourself in the eye, and say you need something to cover it with so you can go to work. Or, you could just try the truth, and when the time comes to purchase more, you'll know exactly where it is. In any case, you've completed step one.

Step two: Pour a small amount onto the makeup wedge, apply where needed. Pat your face dry with a moist towel. Using this method your little jar of foundation should last a long time.

Shampoos

Many shampoos are filled with harsh detergents, oils, parabens (the fancy term for wax), and sulfates, which dry out your scalp and block the pores. This is the reason I believe washing your hair every day is not a good idea. Parabens have been linked to producing estrogen in the body, breast cancer, and accelerating puberty in young women. Most commercial shampoos are loaded with sulfates and parabens, so beware of the so called "natural" shampoo you find in most shops.

When it comes to shampoo, ask the professionals. You might have to pay a little more, but it's worth it. The same goes for conditioners. If you can't afford to spend that much, read the label before you buy. Try to find a shampoo that has a minimal amount of sulfates and no paraben. As a slogan from an old TV commercial used to proclaim, "Only your hairdresser knows for sure!"

Dry Scalp

If you suffer from dry scalp, I highly recommend, Kevin Murphy's Born Again. This product works. Period. (You might want to check out all the other exceptional hair products in the Kevin Murphy line.)

Dry Skin

Once, many years ago, while living in the colder climes, I suffered from eczema. The doctor I went to see told me three magic words, "Moisturize, moisturize, moisturize!" If you have dry or scaly skin anywhere on your body, it simply means your skin is not getting enough moisture. To solve this problem purchase a natural botanical based moisturizer or:

Take a Hot Bath

Now I know this should be in the bathing section, but most of us don't take baths to cleanse ourselves. We do it to relieve stress, soak our weary bones, relieve muscle strain, and to relax for a while from the minutiae of everyday life. A hot bath is extremely therapeutic for your skin. Stay away from bubble-baths, and opt for a sea salt solution when you fill the tub. An array of these products can be had at any Bed, Bath and Beyond, or your local pharmacy. Try to find one without fragrance. If you like, put a few drops of Eucalyptus in the water. This has been known to alleviate aches and pains. Now most bath salts have a tendency to dry the skin out a bit. This works for my type of skin, but if you have naturally dry skin, apply some moisturizer on your body after you're done. Put on some classical music, (I suggest Mendelssohn's String Quartet) and enjoy.

Healthy Diet, Healthy Skin

Avocados are not just for smearing on your face, they contain biotin, which is equally as good for your skin when eaten. So here's a short list of some wonderful foods that will help you have healthy, younger looking skin.

1. Tomatoes. The tomato, besides making great sauce, is a great source of the antioxidant lycopene and is high in carotene. These nutrients may be beneficial in slowing down cellular damage to your skin.

2. Salmon. We all know of the benefits of eating salmon. Those Omega-3 fatty acids help improve skin's elasticity. And it tastes so good.

3. Let's go Nuts. Most nuts also contain Omega-3 fatty acids. Walnuts especially have a higher amount of this nutrient. Some research has shown people who eat nuts tend to live longer, but they go nuts. (A small joke)

4. Eggs. Eggs help in the repair of the skin.

5. Beans. A good source of protein, they create amino acids that help repair skin cells.

So make a nice green salad, and throw in some nuts, avocado, salmon and beans. Squeeze a little lemon juice on top and be kind to your skin.

To lead into my next topic on the subject of Tattooing I will quote the wisdom of my sister Ginger who is fond of saying, "When you get older you want stuff to leave your body." By stuff she means: age spots, wrinkles, spider veins, skin pulls, discolorations, unsightly hairs, etc. I'd like the reader to know that this is just my take. Just my opinion. I'm not passing judgment. I just don't understand this particular trend.

Tattoos

We have all done things when we're young that seemed cool at the time. Some are reversible, and some are not. I had my ear pierced when I was sixteen, and for many years as a Rock n' Roller, I wore it well. I recently tried putting in a small stud just for laughs and honestly, it looked stupid. The difference between a small pin prick through my earlobe and a tattoo is obvious once I removed the earring you would never know it was there. Not so with a tattoo.

When I was a kid, the only people who had tattoos were sailors and hoodlums. I think it's important to state that I'm not anti-tattoo, I know many people who have body art, it's just not my thing, and I realize that this is a more of a lifestyle choice than a fad. But just remember this, you're not going to be twenty-five forever. As you age, your skin loses elasticity. Combine this with the eventual fading of the tattoos, and what was once vibrant and youthful doesn't wear so well when middle age creeps around.

There are a few different methods of tattoo removal. I believe laser removal is the most prominent one. This can be very costly, somewhat painful, and usually leaves a noticeable imperfection of the skin pigment where the tattoo used to live. There are other methods for this process that involve fading lotions applied over a period of time. I don't know how effective these treatments are, so if you go down this path, do your research. Best rule here: If you decide to get a tattoo, keep it simple and out of sight. Refrain from getting any body art on your neck, face, hands and forearms. Allow me to reiterate, if you're a rock star or someone who never had to look for work, fine, knock yourself out. But you don't want to be at a job interview donning your best suit and tie with "Love" and Hate" tattooed on your knuckles, or a scorpion peeking out over the collar of your freshly starched shirt. That's all

3

Mirror, Mirror

One of the first things most people do when they wake up in the morning is go to the loo and look in the mirror. What you see is that most singular part of your person that makes you, you.

No other part of your anatomy says, "This is who I am" more than your face. Next time you visit Mr. Mirror, take a good look. Examine your face. Decide what you like about it and what you'd like to change. I'm not suggesting you run out and see a plastic surgeon (we will cover that option later on) but many imperfections in one's appearance can be changed through better grooming and proper skin care.

It's always amazed me that the one part of our body most people see, we can only view by looking in a mirror. Our faces are truly remarkable with forty-three muscles that are capable of thousands of different expressions. From tears to laughter, pain to elation, a wink to a snarl, our faces tell our emotions consciously and unconsciously, even while sleeping. So let's have some face time.

First thing to do is take a good look at your hair, specifically your hairdo. What kind of hair do you have? Curly, straight, bushy, thick, thin, light, dark? Here are some interesting facts about hair.

1. Hair is the second fastest growing tissue on the body, second only to bone marrow.

2. On average, women's hair is about half the diameter of men's.

3. The anticipation of sex makes hair grow faster. (I guess that's why I seem to be losing mine)

4. By age fifty, over 50 percent of men will have some kind of male-pattern hair loss.

Most men wear their hair short. The upside of this is that it takes very little maintenance to keep it looking good. Decide what you like about your hair, and in what ways you would change it, if any. As young men, we usually wear our hair longer. As we get older, and our hairline starts to recede, we tend to move away from wearing bangs to a more grown up, sophisticated look.

Rule number one:

Spend the money on a good haircut.

I can't emphasize this enough. A ten dollar haircut looks like a ten dollar haircut for a reason. Stay away from chain salons that promise a great cut on the cheap. You might as well put a bowl on your head and do it yourself. Find yourself a great stylist and stick with them.

Do your homework: If you see someone who has a great do, ask them where they had it done. If you're thinking about changing your current hair-style but don't exactly know what you want, buy a copy of G.Q., find something you think might work, and bring it with you when you go to the salon. A good hair stylist will give you an honest assessment, and try their best to make you look good. After all, that's their job, and they want you to keep coming back.

If you're one those unfortunate men who's going prematurely bald, avoid comb overs, toupees and wigs. If you decide to have hair replacement, do some research. Hair restoration can be very expensive, sometimes painful, and honestly it very seldom looks natural. You might want to go with shaving your head completely bald, which is very much in style these days, and considered by some to be very sexy. Think Jason Statham and Bruce Willis.

Avoid blow drying. This is an unnecessary step for short hair and can be damaging over time. Buy a good hair brush. There are a myriad of products for grooming and managing your specific hair style. Once again: ask the professionals, or go to the nearest Walgreens, and ask the nice lady behind the cosmetic counter. If you chose to wear your hair long, a great cut is even more important but will require additional time and maintenance. But if that's your style, and you wear it well, I say *Mazel Tov*.

So whichever way you choose to wear your hair, make it's your own unique statement to fit your own unique personality.

The Beard

In this instance, I'm not speaking about the guy who takes the boss's mistress out on a date, I speak of the hair that grows on your chinny, chin, chin.

For centuries men have worn beards for many different reasons: as a sign of manhood, to protect themselves from the elements, for religious purposes, and to look fierce in battle. But more than likely, shaving with a dagger was tricky business, and probably a royal pain in the ass. Having a long beard in battle wasn't always a plus either. No matter how menacing they looked, many a warrior was held by their beard while their opponent chopped off their head. Eeek! Alexander the Great (356-323 B.C.E.) had enough of this beard pulling business, and ordered all his soldiers to be clean shaven. This new look spread through the empire, and even made its way into Roman times. But the beard lived on in other cultures, and remains to this day. So if you wear a beard, a few tips:

1. A beard will always make you appear older.

2. Unless you're a rock star, independently wealthy, or work in a field where your appearance doesn't matter, steer clear of the ZZ Top, mountain-man look.

3. Pick a style that fits your face.

4. With your magnifying mirror, spend time sculpting your beard.

5. If your beard is going gray, and you're reluctant to shave it off, dye it.

6. Always keep your beard close and neatly trimmed. A good pair of barber shears and an electric trimmer are indispensable for this, and other hair issues.

Which leads us to the next topic:

Shaving

There's a good reason that shower and shave are part of the three S's. For those of you who are not acquainted with the three S's they stand for

Sh#t, Shower, and Shave. My darling niece, at a very young age, came up with a fourth S – Shampoo! But I digress. Showering before you shave does one very important thing: it softens your beard. This is the reason why a barber puts a hot cloth on your face before he shaves you. Most men already know this, and don't need anyone to tell them how to shave their own face, but here are just a few tips.

1. If you're one of those men who doesn't have a full growth everyday (like me) a good electric shaver is a must for those in between days.

2. If you decide to follow the three S's, don't dry your face when you exit the shower.

3. If the can of shaving cream/gel is cold, put it in the sink and run it under hot water for a minute or two. If the shaving cream itself comes out cold, cup your hand and briefly run hot water over your hand. Lather well.

4. Use a good disposable razor. (I know the cartridges are pricey but I will give you a tip on how to make them last longer)

5. After you're finished your initial shave, grab your scissors, hold on to that razor, and take out your magnifying mirror to do some fine tuning. Check under your nose, check your ears, and check your neck. If you see any errant hairs shave them. Remember my friend Bryan at the beginning of this saga, look up your nose, take your trusty scissors, and cut those hairs out!

6. Now, after you're finished with all this, you're going to need an astringent. You could go with an aftershave, but I use Isopropyl Rubbing Alcohol 70 percent, and I use it for everything. Take a paper towel, pour some alcohol on it, and rub your entire face. Then pour some on your razor; it will keep the blade sharp longer.

Eyebrows

Briefly, with your magnifying mirror, take a good look at your eyebrows.

Now, using the small teeth of your comb, brush them away from the center of your face. If you see any unruly hair trim them. For extra-long hairs, take your tweezers and pluck the hair; it shouldn't grow back. If it does, repeat the process.

Manscaping

It seems to be the fashion in these modern times for men and women alike to trim, or shave their genital area. If you decide to do this, best bet is to do it in the shower, with a disposable razor, and tread lightly. In other words: be gentle with your Von Stooker!

4

Apparel

When I was a young lad, and didn't know better, a woman I was seeing asked me if I would accompany her to a social function. I replied in the positive. She then asked if I owned a suit. I replied in the negative. (I told you. I didn't know better)

To wit she said, "Well you better go buy one, because you're not coming with me dressed in dungarees!" (That's what we used to call jeans)

The point of this story is, whether you're young or old, every man should own a few good suits, and the accoutrements that complete the outfit. (Hey, you never know when someone is going to die or get married.) Yet it's surprising how many men I've met in my life who don't care about the way they look, and are content to spend their lives sporting the same old beat-up jeans and leather jacket that went out of fashion with the mullet, platform shoes, and Frankie Goes to Hollywood. I'm guessing if you've make it this far, you're serious about your appearance and looking good, so let's move on to attire. There is a vast array of men's fashion and accessories, but unless you're a model for G.Q., or a total fashionista, a few basic items of apparel should get you through.

As I stated in the introduction, if properly stored and cared for, your wardrobe should serve you well for quite some time. As you become more fashion conscious, your eye for adding to, and updating, your wardrobe will follow suit. (I made a pun.) So let's begin.

An elderly man starts to experience terrific headaches. After a few months of almost daily discomfort, he decides to go see a doctor. After the examination, the doctor tells him the only way to alleviate the pain is castration. The man goes home, speaks with his wife, and after a heartfelt discussion, they decide this is the best course of action. After surgery, the pain goes away, and a few weeks later he was his old self again. One day, while out shopping, he wanders into a haberdashery and says to the salesman behind the counter, "I'd like to buy some underwear; 28 — 30 waist please."

The salesman looks him up and down and states, "Mister, I don't mean to be rude, but I believe you are a 34 — 36 waist."

The elderly man declares, "Don't tell me what size I am, I've been wearing 28 — 30 waist underwear all my life!"

The salesman replied, "Mister if you wore underwear that tight, you'd get terrible headaches!"

The moral of this tale is: Wear Clothes that Fit Properly!

Briefly on Briefs

Whether you sport boxers, briefs, bikinis, or for that matter, boxer-briefs, make sure they're of good quality with an elastic band that's comfortable, and in your size. I know men have a habit of holding on to their underwear way too long. This is not about hygiene, it's about a continued comfortable fit. When the elastic starts to fade, throw them out.

The Shirt

There are many different classifications of shirts, such as casual, polo, and tee, but for now, we will start with the dress shirt. Dress shirts are manufactured in many different fabrics. The one best known to us is cotton or a cotton blend. The optimum word in fabric quality is "thread count." The higher the thread count, the more supple and durable the fabric. A shirt made from Egyptian cotton is generally considered the top of the line, and as you can imagine, tends to be costly. For now we'll stick with the more moderately priced fabrics for everyday and dress wear.

When purchasing a shirt, it's important to know your neck size and arm length. Any salesman worth his weight will be glad to measure you and assist you in finding the right shirt. The label on the inside of the collar will tell the tale.

As an example: 100 percent cotton, 16 ½ neck, 32 — 33 arm length. Now if you need to have a dress shirt for everyday work, you might want to go with a cotton polyester blend. This particular shirt used to be called, "wash and wear" and for the most part, still is.

This type of fabric is easy to maintain and only needs a partial ironing, if at all. Always try to find a shirt that is at least 65 percent cotton. Once again, while in the men's department, ask questions. A good, well fitted shirt doesn't have to cost a fortune.

The Collar

There are many different types of collars. From the cutaway to the button down, from the wing tip tuxedo to the spread. And albeit the style of men's collars has gone from stiffly starched button-on to subtle refinement, I think it's safe to say the collared shirt is here to stay. For now, we will concern ourselves with five basic types.

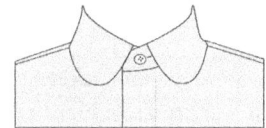

The Club Collar: This particular collar is common with more casual attire, such as golf wear and the like. But it does appear in dress wear, and is usually worn without a tie. I recently saw a rock star at an awards show donning a club with a tie, and he made it work. I suggest not wearing this at a formal function. More *casual cool* than dress up.

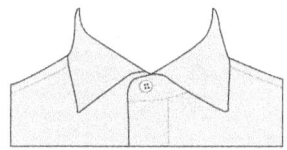

The English Spread: This collar seems to be very popular lately. It's worn with a wide tie, and is personally not my cup of tea. There is a shorter version of this collar that I believe should never be worn with anything other than a bowtie.

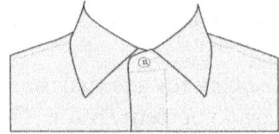

The Spread: Very popular and never out of style, this classic collar can be worn with or without a tie. Extremely versatile, it is well received in black or white, and anything in between, including two-tone.

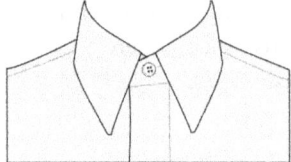

The Pointed Collar: This is the going to a job interview, taking your new paramour to that chic new restaurant, getting invited to a New Year's Eve party at the Metropolitan, attending an upscale dinner gathering with people of renown—collar. Clean, crisp white is preferred. Looks sharp with a beautiful tie, and an equally dashing suit. For formal affairs of all kinds, except when a Tux is required; you can never go wrong.

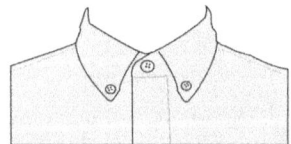

The Button Down: Never starched or stiff, most button down collars are soft and subtle, and never require collar-stays. Great for work when a shirt and tie are called for. Equally at home for weekend fun at the summer house, and walks on the beach with your favorite girl, sans the tie.

Tie Bars (or tie clasps)

Items such as this are a matter of personal taste. There are literally as many different styles as there are ties. Any reputable men's clothing store should have a moderate display, ranging in variety and price. And you can find thousands of different brands online. Depending on what style of tie you prefer, make sure the tie bar will accommodate the width of the tie. You might want to rummage through thrift stores and find that antique gem from the fifties. I have more than a few. They're very retro.

Cuff Links

Somewhere in the course of life, most men are asked to attend a black tie function, or the season premiere of "Le nozze de Figaro." This will require you to wear a French cuff shirt. You will need cuff links. Best rule here: keep it simple, possibly a color that matches your suit. There are thousands of cufflinks available online, and once again, a good men's clothing store will have what you need.

The Suit

My mum used to say, "You can never go wrong with a suit." And she was right. Not to sound cliché, but it's true that first impressions can only be made once.

Suits come in an array of different fabrics: wool, cotton, linen, silk, flannel, and the like. The higher the thread count, the more costly the suit. If you can go out and spend $3,000 on a suit, I say "Mazel Tov!" But if not, here are a few suggestions when it comes to purchasing a suit.

1. Fabric Selection. Of all the fabrics mentioned above, the most common is **wool**. Wool is a durable, breathable, wrinkle-resistant cloth that's easy to maintain, and if properly cared for, should last until the leisure-suit comes back in style. (Hopefully never.) Wool can be worn all year round and will actually keep you cool in the summer.

Cotton is another durable fabric that has the ability to absorb moisture, which keeps you cool, making this a perfect fabric for a summer suit. Also, it's easy to maintain and machine washable, but I don't suggest it.

Linen is a fabric that I feel should only be worn if you live in Key Largo. A white linen suit with a Panama hat looks great, until you sit down. This particular fabric should come with a valet to iron it every half hour.

There is nothing like a **silk** suit, but silk can be costly, and is not intended for everyday use. Silk suits have a sheen that ranges from a shimmer to a subdued polish. If you'd like something in between, go with a wool/silk blend.

2. Look for a sale. We have all seen those endless television commercials that advertise "buy one suit and get two free!" This is a good place to start. For one thing you'll know there will be an army of salesmen eager to make a sale. Since most of us can't afford to have our suits custom-made, having a knowledgeable salesman who measures you correctly, and makes helpful suggestions on fabric choice and style is a big plus.

3. Sizing. When buying a suit off the rack, make sure the suit fits comfortably – not too tight, not too loose, buttons easily, shoulders are straight, and the cuffs and hem are proper length. Tip: The hem of the suit should extend to the palm of your hand. When it comes to your trousers, wear the appropriate shoes. The pants cuff should buckle slightly at the tongue of your shoe.

4. Style. Go with your instincts on this front. Good rule: Purchase at least one dark suit. (Remember the marriage and death stuff?) Know what colors work for you. There's a reason why most women look good: they know the shades of colors that suit their skin type, eyes, and hair. Example: If you're hair resembles Carrot Top's, wearing a bright green suit will make you look like Emmett Kelly. (If you don't know who Emmett Kelly is, think Bozo the clown.)

Pick out a few suit jackets you might fancy and try them on. See how they look. There are a few basic kinds of suits. For instance, single-breasted with one, two, or three buttons, and the double-breasted suit. The three button suit seems to be very popular these days as the double-breasted variety has waned. If you're a little overweight, stay with darker fabrics, and a cut that's slimming, preferably the single-breasted two button. As tempting as it might be to purchase a suit that looks like it's made out of silver, go with something that will stay in style for a bit. For most, you'll know it when you see it. Follow your instincts.

5. Consignment shops and thrift stores. Every once in a blue moon you can find a real gem at the Salvation Army, Goodwill, or your local thrift store. (As long as you don't have a problem wearing something that was worn before.)

Apparel

I love going to the thrift store. Some of the coolest shirts, suits, and especially ties. I've found on my endless journeys scouring the racks of the Salvation Army. If you find a pair of really groovy trousers and don't feel like trying them on, here's a tip my dear friend Mikel gave me: With the button or clasp secure, and the pants zipped up, hold the pants up in front of your waist. Grabbing both ends of the waistband, wrap the pants around your neck. If they fit around your neck in this position, they'll fit your waist. Groovy.

6. Care. Just a few quick tips on care and storage: Always hang your suits on proper hangers; wooden hangers are preferred. Buy a coat brush; brush the suit before and after you wear it. After use, make sure to empty the pockets so as to not to weigh the suit down. (This will cause the jacket to lose its shape over time.)

Leave ample room in your closet to hang suits properly. If your clothes look like they're strangling each other, you don't have enough room. Keep the closet door closed to avoid dust and airborne particles from settling on your clothes. Always dry clean. If your suit or pants become wrinkled, with a cool iron gently press the area, or hang the suit in the bathroom while you shower. If you experience a stain do not use water especially on a light colored fabric. Use only a perchloroethylene based solvent, or take it to a dry cleaners and ask to have the stain removed. If you want to be really punctilious: hang your suits according to color. Not only will this make a specific item easy to find, but it looks nice.

7. Belts and suspenders. Besides style, fit is the most important aspect when purchasing a belt. Know your waist size and get one that fits properly without having to punch an extra hole in the band. Buy a good quality leather belt. The buckle should complement the appearance and color of the trousers you wish to match them to. In other words, don't wear a cowboy buckle on a pair of cuffed gabardines. Belts are meant to be understated. It's not a sash or a cummerbund or a rope, and unless you're Robin Hood, wearing a red belt with green pants is just not done.

Suspenders come in all sorts of colors and fabrics. Once again, match them to the pants and suits you wish to use them on. Stay away from snaps, if you can. The Y-back, button type are preferred for dress wear. If the pants you own don't have the requisite buttons, find a tailor and have them sewn in. Suspenders with elaborate designs and color patterns look clownish, steer clear. (Sorry, Larry King).

8. Be a Beau Brummell. So who was this debonair fellow whose name has become synonymous with stylish dress and elegant grace? His full name was George Bryan "Beau" Brummell, and he was born in Berkshire, England on June 7th, 1778. Educated at the famous Eton School (George Orwell's alma mater) he made his way to Oxford, joined the military, became friends with the Prince of Wales, the future George IV, inherited a few pounds, hung out with the aristocracy, was revered by men, loved by women, and if all that wasn't enough, he single-handedly changed the course of men's fashion forever.

So how did Mr. Brummell accomplish such a leviathan feat? By doing two simple things: He was known to take hours making his morning toilette. He didn't believe in perfume, but instead he was religious about the act of bathing properly and fastidious grooming. So impressed was the Prince with the appearance of the "king of the dandies" that often times he spent hours with him in his loo picking up tips.

Beau was also meticulous when it came to his dress. He rejected the gaudy couture of the higher classes. No hot, bejeweled, sweaty, smelly brocade for this gentleman. His attire was understated and refined. He wore very little jewelry, if any, never donned a wig, chose long pants over knickers, and always wore a cravat (a holdover from his days at Eton, and the precursor to the modern necktie).

The simplicity of his dress was imitated by men of all classes and walks of life. (Too bad he didn't have a press agent, he would have made a bundle!) Much to his chagrin, and those of the snooty class, this allowed the everyday bloke to dress like a gentleman. And in the words of the fictional character, Barry Lyndon, "no outward difference (can be seen) between my Lord and his groom."

Beau was more than a bit of a snob. He was so insouciant, and outright rude, to everyone that eventually he didn't have a friend in the world. As time marched on, Mr. Brummell fell from the good graces of the Regency. He ran up bags of debt, fled England and in 1840, he died broke, alone, and insane from syphilis in an asylum on the outskirts of Caen, France at the ripe old age of 62.

His contribution and legacy to men's attire, and the genteel arts, can't be understated. If it wasn't for Beau Brummell, working guys could still be dressing like stevedores bellowing, "Good day, Gov'ner!"

Cologne

If you decide to wear cologne, two simple suggestions:

1. Go to any reputable department store, find your way over to the cosmetic counter, and spend some time with one of the beautiful young ladies who will be only too glad to suggest something suitable for a man of your caliber. Finding a fragrance that suits you is a very subjective process, so take your time. Good men's cologne can be costly, but if used properly, can last a long time. So spend the money and get something simpatico!

2. Cologne is not aftershave or astringent! Nothing is worse than sitting next to someone who reeks of cologne. (Especially cheap cologne!) The optimum word here is subtlety. Apply your fragrance sparingly. A few light dabs behind your ears or on your neck after a shower should do the trick.

Jewelry and Accessories

I'm of the opinion that when it comes to this particular category, currently referred to in today's vernacular as "bling," less is more. Unlike women, who seem to have a limitless array of baubles and beads, this accoutrement for men should be simple and orderly.

1. The Wristwatch. Depending on your financial status, you really only need two watches, a dress watch and an everyday watch. When it comes to the dress watch, avoid purchasing one that's too ornate. Classic style is always of simple and clean design. Make sure it fits well, feels light, and is comfortable on your wrist. Any local jeweler will be glad to adjust the band at minimal cost.

The everyday watch should be of sturdier stock and can be sportier in style. This will be the watch that, "'takes a lickin' and keeps on tickin,'" harking back to a slogan of yesteryear. Durability should be the number one factor in purchasing this watch, but with so many choices, you can still afford to buy something stylish. Store your watches preferably in a felt lined jewelry box. If battery operated, when not in use pull the setting knob out. This will extend the battery life.

2. Rings and Earrings. When it comes to finger rings, the same rule applies, keep it simple. I will wear one or two rings on my fingers, nothing ostentatious. Stay away from gaudy oversized rings with gems, unless that's your style. Use your own judgment, but make sure it's something that fits your personality. When it comes to earrings, small studs and the non-hanging variety seem to wear better on men. After all, we're not pirates.

Shoes

I once owned a beautiful light blue suit. I tried unsuccessfully to find a pair of blue shoes to match. At every reputable department store and shoe outlet I ventured into, I was greeted with the same incredulous response, "Blue shoes!? We got black and brown, no blue." Now mind you, I wasn't in New York City at this time, so that might have had something to do with it, but still, in contrast to the vast array of women's footwear, men seem to be stuck in the 1920's, and unfortunately for us, the variety and styles of most men's dress footwear is limited.

To be honest, the majority of men's footwear is, in a word...boring! I personally own many pairs of two-tone shoes. It's kind of my thing. But I've had to search far and wide for these gems. With the advent of the world's largest Sears catalogue, the Internet, finding groovy pairs of shoes has become a walk-in-the-park, so to speak. I'm reluctant to go down this path because everything I wear, I want to try on first. But that's just me. So here, dear reader, are a few basic tips on the one item of dress you can't live without (unless you're an aborigine from Fiji)...shoes.

1. Most men don't look at other men's footwear. But women do. Women also notice stuff like dimples. Go figure.

2. The most important factor when purchasing footwear is comfort. Know your size. Try the shoes on. Walk around in them. Make sure they feel snug and inviting. If there's any discomfort, don't buy them, no matter how cool they look.

3. Unless you work at a job that requires you to, don't wear the same type of shoe every day, and don't wear the same shoes all the time. Shoes wear out faster than any other item of dress. Have ample pairs of shoes to be able to change-up your wardrobe. (In this instance, get in touch with your feminine side and go buy yourself some shoes!) If you find a pair that you really like, buy two. You'll thank me later.

4. Always use shoe trees when storing your shoes. This helps the shoe maintain its shape. Also, use a shoehorn when slipping into your favorite oxfords.

Apparel

5. Clean your shoes. Every drug store has a section that sells shoe maintenance products. The days of spit-shining your shoes are over; most can be kept clean with some shoe cream and a soft towel.

6. Wear the appropriate shoes for the style of dress. You wouldn't wear a pair of sneakers with a tux; subsequently, you don't wear dress shoes with a pair of Bermuda shorts. It's always perplexed me when I see a well-dressed man with an incongruous pair of shoes.

7. Find a good cobbler in your neighborhood. Depending on the shoes in question, most can be repaired. Also, most local shoe repair outlets will have a few interesting pair of shoes to sell. The art of shoemaking and shoe repair is something that seems to be passed down from generation to generation. So make friends with the cobbler down the block he'll make your shoes look like new.

A man spends ten years in prison. When he's finally released, the guard gives him back the suit he was convicted in. As he's walking down the street, he reaches into his pocket and finds a ticket from a shoe repair shop in the old neighborhood. Curious to discover what shoes he might have left there so many years ago, he walks in and presents the receipt to the old cobbler behind the counter. The cobbler looks at it, and goes behind a curtain into a back room. Reappearing a moment later, he hands the ticket to the ex-convict and says, "They'll be done next Tuesday."

8. Style. Don't settle for the normal man's shoe. Go online and shop around. When you see something you really like, find out who distributes them in your area. If they cost a little more than you wanted to spend, save your shekels and buy them. And now for the other end of your body.

Hats

Until the 1960's, just about every man alive wore a hat. The hat was not some frivolous accessory worn to impress, it was as much a part of a man's equipage as a good pair of shoes. From the Tricorn to the Top Hat, from the Boater to the Bowler, from the Homburg to the Flat Cap, hats have been with us since the Mayflower. (Even the Pilgrims wore some silly hats if I recall.) So what happened? An old wives tale would have us believe that JFK single handedly killed the hat business, since he was the first president not to don some kind of headgear. (This must have really pissed off Harry Truman.) But whatever the reason, little by little, this wonderfully stylish item has made a reappearance in men's fashion.

There are many different types and styles of hats. And as the saying goes, metaphorically speaking, in a man's lifetime he wears many hats. But for now, we'll stick with a few basic models. Hats are made from many different materials. For the sake of brevity, here are the three most commonly used.

Fur felt is a material made from either beaver or rabbit fur. It tends to be soft and subtle, and somewhat water resistant.

Wool felt (you guessed it) is made from wool. Not as pliable as fur felt, and stiff to the touch, the hats produced from this material tend to be of a lesser quality. Good for a knock-around.

Straw There are a number of different kinds of straw hats, ranging from the scruffy to sublime. Straw hats are only to be worn in the summer, or in a tropical paradise.

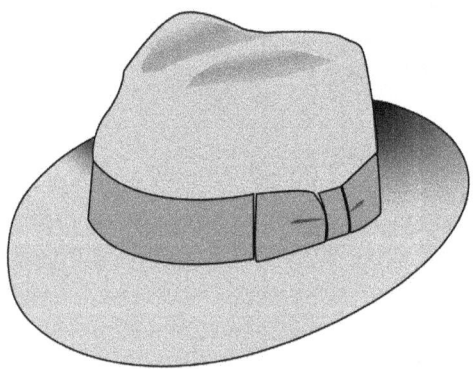

1. The Fedora. Anyone who's ever seen a gangster movie will easily recognize this hat. Worn by criminals and politicians alike, the fedora was by far the single most popular hat of the twentieth century. With its wide brim, and pinched crown, it served the dual purpose of keeping the rain off your shoulders and keeping a low profile.

Apparel

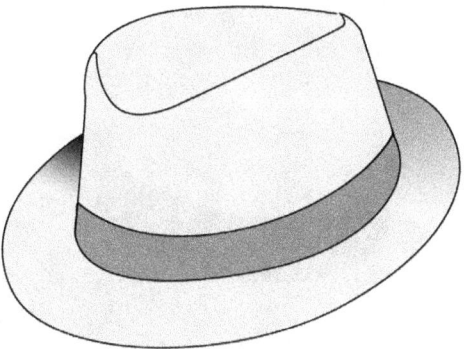

2. The Trilby. Sometimes called the fedora's younger brother, the trilby is basically a fedora with a smaller brim. A much more style oriented hat, it's compact, sturdy, and easy to store. Also called a short brim fedora, I prefer this style over all.

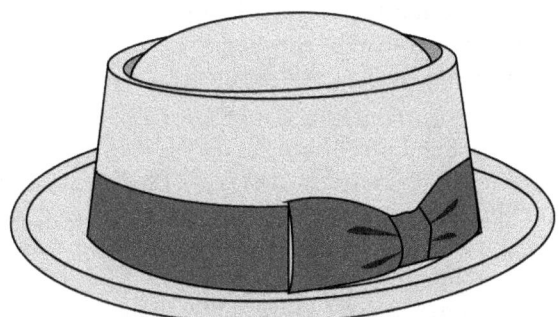

3. The Pork Pie. A pork pie is mostly make from the same material as the fedora or trilby, the difference is that the crown of the hat is oval in shape, somewhat flat, or slightly domed, with a crease running around the inside top edge. The brim is narrow and curled up on the end. Think Gene Hackman in The French Connection.

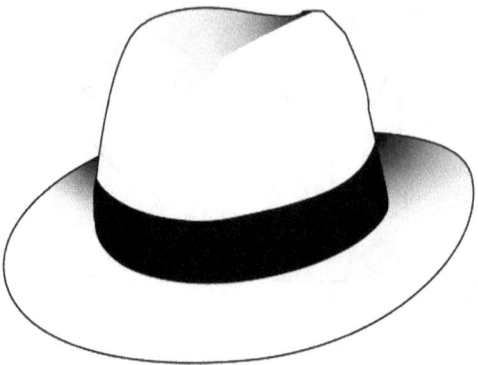

4. The Panama. Strangely enough, the Panama hat was first produced in Ecuador. It seems that the Ecuadorians exported so many of these superbly crafted hats to Panama that after a while, people started calling them "The Panama Hat." They are made from a local plant known as the toquilla palm. A famous photograph from 1904 depicts then President Theodore Roosevelt sitting on a giant steam shovel, wearing a Panama as he inspected the construction of the Panama Canal. This caused its popularity to soar! (Take that JFK.) It was so in demand that the sales of this hat financed a revolution in Ecuador.

This is the perfect warm weather hat. Almost always light colored, the fabric is lightweight and breathable. A genuine Panama hat can be pricey, but it's worth it. The most expensive type of Panama is called Montecristi Superfino, named after the town they're produced in. The same town where Eloy Alfaro Delgado was born and raised, sold a bunch of hats, started a revolution, and became president of Ecuador! That's one impressive hat. So here are a few basic tips about acquiring a hat, and how to care for it, with some hat etiquette thrown in for good measure:

1. *Never buy a hat online.* Unless you're purchasing the exact same product you already have, buying a hat online is a definite no-no.

Start by finding an established haberdashery, or hat shop, in your area. Go there and look around. A real hatter will have a varied selection of different shapes and sizes. Don't start trying on hats indiscriminately. Well-made hats are not some gag item they are as much a part of men's apparel as an expertly tailored shirt.

When you find one that suits you, try it on. If you don't know your hat size, consult the following sizing chart, or ask the hatter. A good hatter can usually tell just by looking at you. If the hat fits, look on the inside at the back of the headband. A small tag will tell the tale; this is your hat size. (I wear a 7 3/8.) Remember this number. When trying on a hat, always handle it by the brim do not grab or pinch the crown.

Take a good look in the mirror from all sides. You might want to try pulling the brim down in front. How does it feel on your head? You want your hat to be snug but not tight. Ask questions. What is this particular style called? What material is it made of? A well-crafted hat should have a silk or similar lining with a leather headband. When you find that special hat that fits your head and your personality, you'll know it. After your purchase, even if you decide to wear your new hat home, ask the hatter for a hat box; you'll need it later. A new hat can make you feel like a new man. You might even start talking like Bogart.

2. Beware of so called, "hat stores" in shopping malls. They usually just sell baseball caps, and a baseball cap is not a hat.

3. Don't be afraid to ask. If you see someone who has a hat that you like, ask them where they purchased it. If you'd like to try it on, ask them. Once again, for serious hat people; a hat is not a toy. If they say yes, and the hat is too small, do not try and stretch it to fit your head. I can't begin to tell you how many times some knucklehead has grabbed my hat, messed with the brim, and stretched it out. In other words; don't mess with my lid! Look on the inside of the hat, all the information is there. On the inside crown is a label that indicates who distributes the hat. On the headband will be the style of the hat, and possibly the store that sells it. Example: Style: Borsalino "Mascot," U.S. Distributor: Dobbs Fifth Ave. Store: Batsakes Cincinnati, OH. (By the by, Batsakes is a wonderful establishment.) If this information isn't there, the hat is probably some wool felt knock-off of inferior quality.

4. Wearing a hat indoors. Here are the rules as I know them: You can wear your hat while sitting at a bar. This is considered acceptable hat etiquette. When sitting at a table, unless it's a card game with your closest associates, you must remove your hat.

5. Always put your hat down on the crown. Placing your hat on its brim will cause the brim to become misshapen over time. Also, always take your hat off by grabbing the side of the brim. Never grab or pinch the crown. If it's just a knock-around, use your own judgment.

6. Cleaning. If your hat gets dirty or dusty, take out your trusty lint brush, and remove whatever debris you can, then with a soft bristle brush, gently brush the hat from front to back. If your hat gets wet, shake it out, then let it dry at room temperature. Once it's dry, repeat the process with the soft bristle brush. If your hat becomes misshapen, for whatever reason, boil some water and with protective gloves on, hold it over the steam and try to shape it by hand. If this doesn't work, take it back to place of purchase and have it re-blocked.

7. Storage. Always store your hat crown down. A good place to keep it is in the hat box you got from the haberdasher. You can also put it on a clean shelf in your closet. You might even want to put it in a small plastic bag to keep the dust off. If it's your everyday hat, a hat rack or solid hook will do.

8. Never put a hat on a bed! This is the worst kind of bad luck. My Aunt Gee Gee told me putting a hat on a bed means death! Granted, an old superstition, but I adhere to it.

9. Hat size chart. With a cloth measuring tape, measure the circumference of your head at the place where you think it might feel comfortable wearing a hat. Take the measurement in inches, and refer to the chart below.

Inches	Hat Size
21	6 3/4
21.5	6 7/8
22	7
22.25	7 1/8
22.75	7 1/4
23	7 3/8
23.6	7 1/2
24	7 5/8
24.25	7 3/4
24.75	7 7/8
25	8

10. My Kingdom for a Hat? Just one more interesting fact: Geoffrey of Anjou, father of Henry II, King of England in 1154, wore a sprig (planta) of broom plant in his hat; hence the name The Plantagenets. This family ruled England for hundreds of years, fought in the Hundred Years' War, and started the War of the Roses. You get the picture. Ahh, the power of the Hat!

5

Etiquette

In 1558, a book was published posthumously entitled *Galateo: Or the Rules of Polite Behavior*. It was written by an Italian, Giovanni Della Casa, an ecclesiastic intellectual, as a guide to his young nephew, Annibale. Unlike Castiglione's *Book of the Courtier* (1528) and Machiavelli's *The Prince* (1532) which dealt mostly with court etiquette and political protocol, Della Casa's book was a guide for the common man. (The period of time in which he wrote is considered by most historians as the beginning of modern man.)

As you can imagine, some of Giovanni's notions on how to be the perfect gentleman are antiquated, outmoded and completely out of sync with our advanced times. For instance, he advises not to wash your hands when returning from the toilet as, "the reason for washing himself will reveal [in other's] imaginations something repulsive" and to "keep your dreams to yourself" as he considered most to be, "by and large idiotic." But many more stand the test of time, and are still relevant today. In a poignant message to his favorite nephew he states, "If those who took care of me in childhood, when we are tender and impressionable, had known how to bend my habits, maybe somewhat hard and coarse by nature, and how to soften and polish them, I could probably have become the man I am trying to make of you."

Galateo was a big hit way back when, and throughout the years it has been referenced by many authors on the subject of Renaissance behavior and more recently by the likes of Emily Post, Judith Martin (Miss Manners) and others in the etiquette field. So dear reader, here are some gems from the sixteenth century. The direct corollary between the days of Michelangelo, Machiavelli, and the Medici to modern times might surprise you.

1. It is improper for a polite gentleman to arrange himself to relieve his physical needs in sight of others. Nor, when finished, should he return to their presence still adjusting himself in his clothing.

2. You must watch your singing, especially solo, if you are tone deaf or sing off key. Few can resist doing this; in fact, it seems the less one's natural musical talent, the more one sings!

3. You do not want, when you blow your nose, to then open the hanky and gaze at your snot as if pearls and rubies might have descended from your brain.

4. When dining, a man of good manners must watch himself that he does not smear his fingers with so much with grease that his napkin is left filthy; it is a disgusting sight.

5. When speaking with someone, do not get so close as to puff on the person's face, for you will find that many do not like to inhale someone else's breath, even though there may be no bad odor.

6. Those who do not care about others' pleasure or displeasure are rude, inappropriate, and unrefined. Therefore, our manners are attractive when we regard others' pleasures and not our own delight.

7. Dress nicely, and according to your status and your age. Clothes must also fit well and suit the individual.

8. Arrogance is nothing but a lack of respect for others; everybody wishes to be respected even if he does not deserve it.

9. Men who are affable and polite will appear to have friends and acquaintances wherever they go. For this reason, it usually behooves you to greet, chat, answer gracefully, and treat everyone like your neighbor or friend.

10. Nothing comes out of the mouths of some others except stories about their children…"Last night my kid really made me laugh!" "You will never see a cuter baby than my little Momo…You wouldn't believe she's as smart as a whip already!" No one has so little to do that he has the time to respond or even pay attention to such rubbish, and so it exasperates everyone.

11. Liars not only are not believed, they are not listened to, like those people whose words lack substance, and whose speech is pretty much blowing hot air. Others forge lies in their own favor, boasting and bragging about great accomplishments or knowledge, aggrandizing themselves, claiming to be brilliant and capable of marvelous deeds.

12. We should neither boast of our advantages, nor make a joke of them, for the one is to reprove others for their shortcomings, and the other is to undervalue their virtues.

13. One should not speak ill either of other men, or of their affairs; of those bad-mouths, figure that what they tell us of others, they could also tell others of us.

14. On giving advice: This should not be done with everyone you know, but only with your best and closest friends.

15. One should never mock a person, no matter how much he is an enemy, for it seems that ridicule shows greater contempt than injury; joking is done for amusement, and mocking is done to harm.

16. Where your pleasantries are not rewarded with the laughter of listeners, cease and desist from telling jokes in the future.

17. Both in polite conversation, and in other types of speech, words must be clear enough that everyone listening can easily understand them, and be equally as beautiful in sound, as in sense.

There you have it; a small smattering of wisdom from a bygone age. And albeit social mores change with the passing of time, many of the initial concepts concerning societal and behavior protocol put forth by *Galateo* still apply. So taking a page from history, and my old paisano, Della Casa, I humbly submit my own apperception learned through many years of trial and error, and making a total fool of myself! on how to present oneself in polite society.

Try to Always be a Gentleman

Politeness and courtesy towards all those around you is part of the tenable structure of civilized society. A simple "thank you" or "I really appreciate your time" can go a long way in life.

Be courteous to everyone you meet. Condescension is the symptom of a narrow mind. No matter what your status in life; whether prince or pauper, everyone deserves respect. Everyone has a story to tell. Look people in the eye when you converse.

John Bradshaw, a wonderful humanist and teacher, is fond of saying, "if everyone did one good deed a day the world would be a better place." I totally agree. During the unpleasantness of an occasional disagreement, taking the high road when dealing with the opposite sex (or anyone for that matter) is always the best course of action. Walking away, and waiting for cooler heads to prevail, is something most men, including me, take some time to grasp. After all, we are men, and it's our nature to defend ourselves. But for now, we'll take a lesson from Shakespeare who advises us that in times like these, "Discretion is the better part of valor."

Dress Appropriately for Every Occasion

It never ceases to amaze me what some people wear when they're out in public. While shopping at a local market recently, I noticed a middle aged, Rubenesque woman sporting an outrageous attire of nothing more than a faded pink sweatshirt and an equally worn pair of matching sweatpants. What was most disturbing about this image was the extremely obvious fact that this woman wasn't wearing any underwear. To put it as genteelly as possible: all her stuff was hanging out!

Now to be honest, we somewhat expect this slovenly behavior to be more prominent amongst men. Especially married men who seem to, at some point during their matrimonial sentence, acquiesce to letting their wife dress them (which sometimes isn't a bad thing). Or they just give up altogether and walk the aisles of Walmart in a pair of broken flip-flops, an ill-fitting pair of torn jeans, a washed-out baseball cap to cover an eight-dollar haircut, and a t-shirt that proclaims, "I'm with Stupid." I'm not suggesting you wear a suit and tie while grabbing a quick snack at the 7-11, (at times like these comfort is the overriding factor) but boarding a plane to go on a trip looking like you just came in from raking the leaves, in my opinion, gives the impression of total apathy, disdain, disregard for social decorum, or just plain stupidity.

You would think that with diverse occasions such as job interviews, weddings, and barbecues the mode of dress would be self-evident, but you would be wrong. (Not to *wax nostalgic*, but let me reiterate that this is the opinion of someone who grew up in a time when people got dressed up to go to the movies, and mothers did their shopping in high heels and spring dresses.) So here dear reader are some subtle suggestions on the do's and don'ts of appropriate attire:

1. Job Interviews. You would think this would be a no-brainer, but depending on the employer, most job interviews are no longer a single meeting with the person in power; they have become a process that involves numerous visits and sit-downs. If your wardrobe is not that extensive, you might find yourself coming up short, but if part of this process is a job-fair or fact finding mission, a more casual look is fine. Save your spiffy suit for the actual interview. If you only have one suit, try wearing a different colored shirt and tie or different dress pants with the same jacket. Bottom line is, when you finally get to see Mr. or Mrs. Big, look your sharpest.

2. Dining. If someone invites you to a barbecue, you're most definitely not going to wear a suit and tie, so why would you wear your barbecue clothes to a dinner party? To do this, unless with very close friends, is to show total disrespect for the host and their dinner guests. At the very least, wear a collared shirt and a sports jacket.

3. Weddings and Formal Affairs. This one is easy: Rent a good tux or wear your best suit.

4. The Beach or Pool. A good friend of mine went to a nude beach with his wife, and when I asked him how it was he said, "All the people you wanted to see naked weren't, and all the ones you didn't, were." Good rule here: If you're not a swimsuit model and a little out of shape like most, avoid wearing a speedo. Some well-fitted swim-trunks with a light short-sleeve summer shirt and a hat should do the trick. After all, you don't want to frighten the children.

5. First Date. This one all depends on where your first date will take place. Assuming you already know that, this should be easy. If going to dinner, a cool pair of jeans, sports jacket, and an open-collared shirt should suffice. Many times the woman in question will ask what to wear, this alone will give you a clue. Subsequently, whatever the circumstance, it never hurts to ask the same question.

6. Vacations/Trips. Next month I will be traveling to New York for a few days to attend a wedding. That tells me I will need two bags: a suit bag for my tux and sport jackets, and a carry on. When going on a trip, most people tend to over-pack. This is unnecessary. The "less is more" rule was never more apropos, so pack light and have a great time.

7. Funerals/Wakes. Simply put: dark suit, black shoes, white shirt, and dark tie –The end.

The Noble Lie

Whether you like it or not, we all lie. Yet everyone we've ever known has uttered the phrase, "be honest with me." In most cases, honesty with a friend or family member is easy. In affairs of the heart, it becomes slightly more complicated. Go to any dating website and you'll find "honesty" high on the checklist of basic wants. We are never 100 percent honest with anyone.

Personally I think honesty is overrated. Trust is much more valuable. So when is it copacetic to lie? If I'm in a relationship with someone for a number of years, I trust that person will always have my best interests in mind, and I theirs. If, during the course of our time together, "Lulu" has a one-time fling with Raul the pool man, I don't want to know. Granted, omitting the truth is not quite the same as lying, so allow me to pose this: Once, while managing a local bistro, a woman whom we'll call Carol was very interested in dating me. She was a short, full-figured woman with a pleasant demeanor, but as a romantic interest, just not my type. Rather than tell Carol I just wasn't attracted to her, I lied. Not a white lie but a noble lie. What purpose would honesty have served then? There's a reason the adjective "brutal" often appears before the word "honesty."

Always Put the Toilet Seat Down

In all cases, this is simply proper etiquette. It especially applies if you're living with a woman or staying at her pad. The unearthly cries of a woman falling in the toilet at 2:oo in the morning are nothing compared to the deafening silence that follows for the next two days, trust me.

Be Chivalrous

In days of old, when Knights were bold, practicing the art of Chivalry was quite the arduous enterprise, and becoming a knight wasn't an easy task. The first requirement was to be born of aristocratic stock. After years of being a page, then a squire and basically a lackey to another knight, you were led into a church where a priest heard your confession, dressed you up in armor, sprinkled holy water on you, and chanted some jazz in Latin. He then tapped you on the shoulder with a sword, and sent you out into the world to find a crusade where you could kill, rape, and pillage.

As a knight, you swore an oath to speak the truth, defend the church, protect the poor, pursue the infidels, be a guardian to all women (preferably Christian women), and to be a brother to all other knights in mutual courtesy and aid. Unfortunately, most knights never followed this code, and basically did whatever the hell they wanted. When there wasn't a crusade to be fought, knights fought each other in tournaments. The reward for these sometimes deadly mock battles and jousts was a kiss from a fair maiden. Seems like a long way to go for a kiss. Nevertheless, the underlying theme of all this pomp and pageantry was "Courtly Love."

In and about the late 1100's, a chaplain named Andreas Capellanus composed a treatise on courtly love. In it he says, "Love teaches everyone to abound in good manners." This was the embryonic beginning of man's transformation from brutish galoot to the refined gentleman of today. Albeit, it only took a thousand years. According to the late, brilliant historian, Will Durant, "modern politeness is a dilution of medieval chivalry."

So now that you know all this, achieving chivalry in our modern world should be fairly easy, and you don't have the cumbersome chore of putting on armor, or mounting a steed. Now some of these acts may seem antiquated and old fashioned, but I believe that a vast number of women still respond to these simple courtesies in a positive way.

1. Buy her flowers. I've never met a woman who didn't like flowers. Try to find out what kind of flora she likes beforehand. If you get to know her family over time, buy her mother flowers. Couldn't hurt.

2. Kiss her hand. Imagine you're a late eighteenth century Count, and go for it. The key to performing this maneuver properly is always bend down to kiss the hand, never grab the hand and bring it to your lips.

3. Write her poetry. If you can't think of anything to write, buy a book of sonnets and read to her. "For thine sweet love remembered such wealth brings, I dare to change my place with kings."

4. Cook her dinner. Most of the great chefs in the world are men, so this is in your DNA. You'll know what culinary fare she likes after a few dates.

5. Sing her a song. If you're really crazy for her, go to her house, bring that old guitar sitting in the corner and sing a song under her window.

6. Always open the door. Whether it's your car, or the door to a restaurant, always allow her to enter first. Subsequently, when taking her home always walk her to her door. And if she drove to meet you always walk her to her car.

7. Help her with her coat. I can't tell you how many times, especially in colder climes, I've witnessed some poor woman struggle with putting on her overcoat, while some young turk stood idly by and offered no assistance. Even if it's a stranger, gently come to their aid. Also, while strolling in the park, if you notice the woman you're with rubbing her arms, take off your jacket and wrap it around her. Don't wait to be asked.

8. Defend her honor. Women like to feel protected. In a social setting, during polite conversation, if the woman you're with poses a different point of view that you agree with, come to her defense. If you don't agree, defend her right to say it.

So there you have it. Chivalry is not dead. And keep in mind that till this day, some women still refer to their man as, "my knight in shining armor."

Be Organized

You remember the last time an acquaintance picked you up in his car, and spent twenty minutes taking all the crap off the front seat, then throwing it on more crap in the back, all the while saying, "I've been meaning to clean this, but I just haven't had the time to get to it!" In a word...bullshit.

Unfortunately, in life some people are just slobs. To me nothing is worse than going to someone's home, and finding it in total disarray and chaos, while the person in question makes some lame joke about the cleaning lady's day off. Everyone has a choice: to be neat and organized or be relegated to making excuses as to why the dishes have been in the sink for a week.

Now you may think that Mr. Sal has always been a fastidious neat freak who never lived in a cluttered room, or threw his clothes on the bed, but you would be wrong. As a young lad, living in the city, playing music, chasing chicks, and partying into the wee hours, my room sometimes looked like a Goodwill box blew-up in it. (Although I always made my bed, and do to this day, for fear my mother may come back from the dead and smack me.) As I got older and gained more insight into life, the benefits of being well-ordered and organized became self-evident.

It's truly astonishing how much stuff, even as a single man, one acquires during a lifetime. Some people I know have accumulated so many belongings and paraphernalia that the classification of "Hoarder" may apply. Here's the bottom line: unless you're one of the Vanderbilts, or a member of the Fortune Five-Hundred, and have a palatial mansion where a biographer archives your precious mementos for posterity, when you die most of your possessions will either be donated, given away, or thrown in the trash. Boo hoo hoo. Such is life. Pardon my redundancy, but once again, "Less is More."

Most of the items that you acquire over the years serve only as an impediment to living an orderly life. The less stuff you have, the easier it will be to keep it clean and organized. Learn to throw things out. Go through your clothes every year. Got a t-shirt, dress shirt, or shoes you never wear? Donate it. Old worn-out paperbacks from your senior year? Throw them out!

A stack of old magazines you never got around to reading? Garbage.

Unless you save your household bills for tax reasons, buy a shredder and make confetti. Worn-out bed sheets and towels? Cut them up and use them to clean. Photos from your adventures in Las Vegas before the internet? Scan them to your computer and throw the hard copies out. A beat-up boom box that doesn't really work anymore? Recycle. A crappy candy dish your Aunt Sadie gave you before she died ten years ago? Throw it in the trash. (Hey, she'll never know.)

Look in your refrigerator, is there a jar of mayonnaise that's turning into a science project, or a take-out container of Indian food that's growing hair a few steps away from the garbage pail? Are there pots and pans in your cabinets that look like they could be useful on a wagon train? When it comes to consolidating your gear, here's a suggestion: go to any drug or hardware outlet and purchase a few plastic storage containers. Make three piles: definitely keep, maybe, and garbage. Whatever you don't immediately need in your home, but want to keep, pack it neatly in a container and store it.

Put the "maybe" pile in a separate container so you can go through it at a later date (and make sure that you do!) And the rest you guessed it—garbage! You'll be amazed how much better you'll feel when you are neat and organized. And if that is not enough to convince you, try this on for size: You meet some groovy, good looking chick and she says, "Let's go back to your place." You'll have two choices: either make up a lie that your pad is being remodeled or say, "Let's go!" You decide.

The Art of Conversation

Verbal communication of the human species is most likely at the heart of every great discovery and advancement in human history. It is interesting to note that neither Socrates, nor the prophet Mohammed, were able to write, so their teachings were handed down verbally to be transcribed at a later date. Such is the power of the spoken word.

Now there are many different kinds of conversation, and verbal intercourse takes on many different forms, depending on who you are speaking to. Your communications with a prospective employer vary greatly from your chit-chat with the check-out girl. And I very much doubt that if you had the honor of meeting the president, or a head-of-state, you would blurt out "Hey, my man, what's up?" In the warm embrace of family and close friends, yakin' at a thousand words a minute, telling racy jokes, and interrupting your guests to tell of your adventures while pouring yourself another glass of vino is usually acceptable behavior, but not so amongst strangers.

If by chance you get invited to dine with your new paramour's parents, or a group of people you just met, a good rule is to qualify your company. The late, great comedic genius, George Carlin, advises us to listen first and see what kind of language is acceptable. If your new girlfriend's mother says the word "shit" during polite conversation, then you know that the word, "shit" is not going to get you banned from their home. That is not to say that you should use such language, but as least you'll have a handle on what is, and is not, welcome.

In the past I've made many a *faux pas* in mixed company with my choice of words. Unfortunately for me, growing up in a city where the "F" word is used in every possible variation thereof, I was startled by the underscored displeasure and shock of many at my use of the word. Overtime, I've learned to qualify the people around me and to discriminate my use of vulgarity. Or I simply said, "F#@k them if they can't take a joke!" (Spoken like a true New Yorker). Which leads us to our next linguistic travail.

1. How to tell a joke. There are a few basic rules on the art of joke telling. The first is the kind of joke to tell. After qualifying the social setting you're in, the nature of your comedic tale will make itself known. In other words, you're not going to tell a joke about the priest, rabbi and minister who wander into a bordello to a bunch of nine-year-olds, and subsequently, jokes about death or dying may be deemed a bit inappropriate to someone's ninety-year-old grandmother. If you've got a hip adult crowd, well versed in the ways of the world, and not adverse to ribald humor laced with a sexual-innuendo or two, let fly. But know this: really dirty jokes are usually not funny, so be selective.

If you don't know any jokes...buy a book. The second part of successful joke telling is knowing the joke, inside and out. I can't begin to tell you how many times while working at a bar I heard someone say, "I've got a joke" and then they proceed to fumble through, "Let me think....oh, I know...two guys walk into a bar and...oh, that's not right...let me start again...a guy goes into a bar with his horse and the bartender says...oh, wait that's another joke...." Blah, blah, blah.

Another kind of bad joke teller is the one who tells a joke with a really small punch line, and takes thirty minutes to get there. Boring! Try to get to the punch line as quick as possible.

This rule also applies to storytelling on the whole. The object is for everyone to still be awake by the end of your narrative. Also, if you can, tell the joke standing up. (They don't call it stand-up comedy for nothing) If you get interrupted for more than a brief moment while telling a joke, the joke, no matter how hilarious, is going to bomb. So don't continue. Never ask if someone has heard a particular joke. If they're polite, they'll let you tell it anyway. And if you've heard a joke someone is telling, never, ever step on their punch-line.

A few years ago, a research group in England did a study on humor, and what makes certain people laugh. They found that men like jokes with aggressive punch lines, whereas, women prefer ones that are more pun or wordplay based. This is also something to consider when telling a joke in mixed company. And if your joke bombs, it means either you told it wrong, it's a bad crowd, or it's a crappy joke. So work on your delivery, and if it fails to get a laugh the second time around, get a new joke. I got a million of them.

A man goes to prison (stop me if you've heard this one...just kidding). On his first day, the entire populace is led into the mess hall, and after lining up to get food, the hall falls into a din of men stuffing their faces. A prisoner jumps up from his seat and yells, "54!"

The whole place bursts out in laughter. A few minutes later another jumps up and proclaims, "37!"

Once again the entire group explodes in laughter. Back in his cell, the new prisoner asks his cellmate what was going on. The old, hardened con explains that in jail they don't hear many new jokes, so they've given them numbers, then they simply say the number and think of the joke. So the con proceeds to tell his new cellmate a few jokes, a few numbers, and a few days later they're back in the mess hall. An inmate jumps up in the back of the room and yells, "44" the place goes wild.

So the new guy decides to try one, he stands up and bellows, "27!" Nothing, the place is dead silent. Once again he yells, "16!" and once again, nothing. He sits down, turns to his cellmate and says, "What happened?"

The cellmate replies, "It's the way you told the joke."

2. Religion and Politics. Anyone reading this who's old enough to drink has had the experience of being at a bar or tavern where the innkeeper or bartender will say of conversation, "No Religion or Politics." There is a good reason for this, especially in mixed company. These two volatile subjects bring out the very worst in people and should only be attempted in the company of intimates. No matter what your religious or political stance may be, unless you're with people of like mind, you're bound to insult someone. If you're ever in this situation where others are engrossed in a heated discussion concerning politicians or prophets, try to change the subject. (Hey! tell a joke.) Also, if you work with someone who constantly tries to engage you in this banter, simply say you don't have an opinion and walk away.

3. You've Got your Troubles, I've Got Mine. Very few, if any live a trouble- free life. This is the exact nature of life itself. Always changing, in constant flux, we all have our ups and downs. And when we do, most of us look to garner sympathy and guidance from our closest friends and family. Usually this is the normal course most of us take. More than likely, we've all been on one side or the other at some point. But no matter how much people might care for you, after a short time of hearing nothing but laments, complaints and self-recriminations, the simple act of speaking with you becomes a tedious and arduous task that most would like to avoid.

I've been guilty of this social *faux pas*, only realizing it when people stopped returning my calls. In my embarrassment, and with the help of a dear friend, I got help and learned a valuable lesson. No one wants to hear you moan and groan, even your family. So if you have problems in your life and get invited to a party, as they say, leave your troubles behind. Nobody wants to hear them. Try and keep your conversation upbeat and lively.

4. Be Yourself. One of the absolutes in life is no matter how nice or positive you are, not everyone is going to like you. That's just the way it is. For whatever reason, there's always going to be someone you rub the wrong way. This should in no way impede you from being yourself during the course of polite conversation. As long as your verbal intercourse is informative, animated, and dynamic, the curmudgeonly demeanor of one dour individual means nothing. If the person in question tries to bait you, politely excuse yourself and mingle.

5. Mnemonics. We're all guilty of this *solecism. You meet someone new, and five minutes later you've forgotten their name. The reason is simple. Most of us are a bit self-centered, and we can't wait to show everyone how special we are. In our haste to make new friends, we forget to listen when being introduced. Now granted if you're introduced to ten people at once, very few of us can rattle off their names later on. But when meeting one or two folks at a time, here's the trick, look the person over and find something about them that stands out. Let's say you meet a guy named "Fred" who just happens to have red hair. Make up a rhyme, Fred the Red. (I know that's an easy one.) How about a woman named "June" who has striking blue eyes. Create a mental picture and say, "June Blue Eyes." If you happen to know the occupation of the person, let's say Paul is a plumber, simply call him Paul the Plumber. I promise if you do this, you'll remember the names of most of the people you meet.

Also, here's something I've done for years. Every woman I was ever involved with I told them this; if we meet someone and I don't introduce you, it means I don't know their name so please put it on me, and say something like, "Sal has no manners, my name is Karen, what's yours?" In return, I will do the same for you. Works out great. (About the only thing that did between me and Karen.)

*a grammatical mistake in speech or writing, a breach of good manners; a piece of incorrect behavior.

6. High Society. When I was a young lad, I sometimes found myself in the company of people from a completely different social status. Most of the time, they treated this street kid with kid gloves, but every once in a while, some condescending, stuffy, old blowhard would use his Ivy League education as a weapon of superiority, and take advantage of a naïve, trusting youth from the streets of Queens. Flashing around twenty-dollar words and discussing events far beyond my scope, I often felt their goal was simply to belittle me for the sake of their own aggrandizement. Usually, my first instinct was to take the person in question out to an alley and throw him a beatin'. (I told you I was a street kid)

As time went on, I learned the best course of action with persons of this ilk is to placate them. That is not to say don't stand-up for yourself, but this sort of hubris can only be defeated with deferment. I am fond of saying that I can hold a conversation with anyone, on any subject, and if asked my views on a subject or topic I don't know enough about, I simply say, "I don't have enough information to give a decisive opinion." If someone uses a word I don't know, I'm not afraid or embarrassed to say, "I don't know what that word means, enlighten me." If during polite conversation, someone poses a fact that you know is incorrect, gently call them on it. If they make an issue of it, don't be deterred from proving them wrong. This open, and hopefully friendly, exchange of ideas is what makes the world go round.

In the end game, words are very powerful. They define in some ways who we are and what we stand for. They should never be used to hurt or demean someone. Their purpose is to enlighten and illuminate the world around us. So speak, listen, and learn; use words wisely.

Here in My Car

It's truly astonishing how brave and angry people get when driving their cars. Put a few inches of steel and an airbag between a person and the road, and suddenly they become "Mad Max." Driving is a learning process, and in these days of super highways and 75 mile-an-hour concrete corridors that seem to stretch to the sun, driving can be an extremely stressful, anxious activity. Couple that with endless traffic jams, bad weather, road construction, the occasional traffic ticket, and it's no wonder that sometimes people flip-out! It's like the weather. When you get into your auto, there is absolutely nothing you can do about these unforeseen issues that impede us all from getting where we need to go. Now let's be honest. Very few of us started off as great, proficient drivers. We're all guilty at some time or another of inadvertently cutting someone off, or of daydreaming, when the light has changed. But as time goes on, and we become much more skilled in the art of motoring, we seem to forget that at one time we were that young kid getting on the highway for the first time with a father yelling, "Give it more gas, speed up, put your blinker on!" We also fail to acknowledge that someday we will be that old man or woman peering through the steering wheel, doing thirty five miles-an-hour in a sixty five mile zone.

As frustrating as it is to be on the receiving end of those who have not yet become, "Masters of the Road," or others who don't care about the drivers around them, leaning on your horn and yelling out the window, or giving people the finger (which I personally think is extremely vulgar) serves absolutely no purpose whatsoever. It does nothing but exacerbate the situation. Now granted, there are those who simply do not pay enough attention when driving, these are the most dangerous, and you should learn to identify them and keep your distance, but I digress. Here are some tips on proper driving etiquette:

1. Always signal your intent. It is important to let other drivers and pedestrians know exactly where you're headed. This is a personal gripe of mine. It is one of the very first instructions I learned, and to this day, I always signal. (Sometimes I point to where I'm going.)

2. Let people get in front of you. When stopping at a light, or pulling out of a parking lot, be noble and let people cut in front of you. It's a small courtesy, and when someone does it for you, give them a wave.

3. If someone cuts you off... Someone cutting you off on the highway can be a very dangerous three seconds. After your heart stops racing, and you're finished thanking the Road Gods, speeding up to find the culprit who caused you all this distress is a lesson in futility.

4. Beep-Beep. Never lean on your horn unless positively necessary. When waiting at a traffic light, if the driver in front of you has fallen asleep, wait a few seconds, and then tap your horn gently. Beep-beep.

5. The Good Samaritan. When driving down the road (not the highway), if you come across another motorist who's stuck, (if time permits) stop and lend a hand. You'll feel wonderful, and will have done your good deed for the day.

The Invitation

If you get invited to an acquaintance's or friend's home, a good rule is to always bring something with you. Arriving with a bottle of wine or some cheesecake shows your appreciation and respect. In my experience this always makes a good impression. If dating a woman, and meeting her parents for the first time, the decision on what sort of item to bring is even easier. Just ask the girl.

Nectar of the Gods.

An ancient Greek, whose name eludes me now, once said, "No civilization can exist without some form of narcotic." The "narcotic" he spoke of is still around to this day. Allow me to state upfront that I make no moral assertion, or cast aspersions, on one's personal drinking habits, and fully understand that most of us who are old enough to drink have, at one time or another, gotten smashed, and probably made fools of ourselves. But for most, having a few drinks with friends is no big deal, and responsible behavior will serve you well in the company of strangers.

Just because I suggested to bring some libations with you when you get invited to someone's home doesn't mean you have to finish it yourself. If you're meeting a group of people for the first time, and want to make a good impression, getting "soused" is definitely not a good idea, no matter how much nectar is flowing. Grace and decorum seem to leave the room when inebriation enters. Anyone who's ever been around a drunk friend or relative can attest to that. Della Casa advises, *"...temperance [will never] be learned from such teachers as wine and intoxication."*

Never take Liberties

This unique, wonderful world we live in is made up of many different, and equally unique, groups of people. Growing up in a city represented by 178 of these diverse multitudes, I've had the pleasure of meeting, and becoming friends with, folks from all different backgrounds and ethnicities. But only with true and lifelong intimates did I ever breach the social contract and jokingly poke fun at their natural origin. This is just not done in polite society. Yet with all this diversity, I always thought of myself as "just a guy from New York," and it wasn't until I ventured out in the world that my specific ethnic background was brought to my attention.

I can only guess at the number of times total strangers have uttered phrases like, "So Sal, you're Italian, right? Are you in the Mafia?" or, "You must be in witness protection if you're here." Most of the time, I let it roll off my back, but that doesn't mean it doesn't bother me, and there have been times I've called people on it by simply saying, "I really don't appreciate that."

An African-American friend of mine who works in the hotel industry says it's amazing how many guests take the liberty of calling him, "Bro." It is tantamount to approaching a stranger in a wheelchair and calling him, "Wheels." In defense of some, I believe they are trying to be affable, not realizing that these sorts of comments are actually hurtful. We are a land of immigrants, and most are trying to blend in and become part of the American fabric. Believing that it's somehow ingratiating to constantly bring to the forefront one's natural origin is misguided at best, and only enhances the possible spread of more division. So don't do it, and don't let others do it to you.

You Gotta Have Friends.

Friendship, next to family, is probably one of the most important things in our lives. During the course of our lives, we meet many people, but very few of them become true friends. It's great to have acquaintances, but a few loyal, trustworthy friends are worth their weight in gold. I've personally been blessed to have a solid group of comrades who forgive me my endless yakin' and pontificating. They have helped me through rough times and celebrated with me when times were good. That is the essence of friendship.

A friend is someone who accepts another's shortcomings. We all have them, as none of us is perfect. So be kind to your friends, listen to what they have to say, take and give advice when asked, stick with them through good and bad, and remember the line from the movie, *It's a Wonderful Life*. "No man is a failure who has friends." Thanks, Clarence.

This is the Modern World

Ah! Cell phones, iPads, wrist phones, personal computers, laptops, e-mails, Facebook – all wonderful, amazing gadgets of modern technology! What would we do without them? Speak to each other more? Read a book? Write someone a letter and physically put in the post? That would be nice. I know I'll probably catch some flak for saying this, but these so-called personal accessories that we can't seem to do without, and for some seem to be welded to their bodies, are in the hands of many the most impersonal and unsociable devices ever invented.

Now, I fully understand the convenience of being able to call or text someone from anywhere in the world at a moment's notice. I, too, enjoy this luxury. But the next time I'm speaking to someone and they're texting while I'm trying to communicate with them, I just might grab the cell from their paws and stomp it to pieces! And why do some folks think it's appropriate for you to hear their entire phone conversation when out in public, especially indoors? When this happens, I usually take out my cell phone, make out like I'm calling someone, then get as close as possible to Mr. Loudmouth and speak at an even higher volume, sometimes mimicking his words and actions. I just think this is extremely rude behavior. There is absolutely no reason to be glued to your phone every minute of the day.

6

The Man Rules

In the year 550 B.C.E., in Ephesus, a city of Ancient Greece, lived a ribald poet of pointed wit named Hipponax. By all physical accounts he was short, thin, lame, and possibly deformed. Not quite the youthful Adonis we've come to equate with the culture that gave us Heracles (Hercules). Nevertheless the Greeks loved his crass, raffish poetry, and Hipponax managed to lead a pretty good life. He's quoted as saying, "Women bring two days of happiness to a man, one when he marries her, the other when he buries her." A misogynistic statement even in those times, considering the fact that the ancient Greeks revered women.

A few years ago, while sitting with a male acquaintance of mine over lunch, he confided in me he was having problems of the heart concerning his recent love interest. More than a few years his junior, the lady in question was making him crazy. He said the sex was great, but everything else paled by comparison. He couldn't quite figure out what was going through her mind. To wit I replied, "Don't even try."

He then sighed and lamented, "You know Sal, when it comes to women there are only two good days in a man's life, the day he meets her, and the day he leaves her."

And there it was, Hipponax reborn! Mind you I totally disagree with this point of view. I happen to find women delightful. But what amazed me is the fact that this quotation, in one form or another, has been around for 2500 years passed down from one generation to another, from brother to brother, father to son.

My father, a man of considerable wisdom, also had a saying for everything. His lexicon of quotations included such gems as, "We'll cross that bridge when we get to it." " It's a great life if you don't weaken," and my childhood favorite, "Don't make me get up!" He was also known to periodically blurt out, "They should have killed those goddamn Beatles, they started this hippie crap, and they brought the drugs over from England." Yes my father was a laugh a minute.

Of all my father's astute observations of the human condition, the one that applies here, and is most apropos, is "If I live to be 150, I will never understand women!" Truer words were never spoken. Men have a better chance of understanding quantum physics, than the feminine psyche. That is not to say that we don't try. Even during REM sleep, our minds are constantly drawn to the female enigma. Every woman we meet poses a new set of variables. The parameters are in a constant state of perpetual flux. Women send out so many mixed messages that if it weren't for the primordial need to have sex, none of us would ever get laid. So here, dear reader, are a few rules to follow that have been handed down through the ages. If you wish to add to this list, be my guest. Our gender can use all the help we can get.

1. Never start an argument with a woman who has a knife in her hands.

(Or any sort of sharp object for that matter.)

2. Never go out with anyone who has more problems than you do.

This happens to be an incredibly good rule which applies to everyone. Here's my theory; we all have stuff we *have* to do: go to work, to school, pay our bills, take out the garbage, walk the dog, shovel the snow, mow the lawn, etc. You get the picture, the everyday vicissitudes of life. So why add more difficulty to your already hectic world by dating someone who's a drama queen?

3. Never confide in your girlfriend's girlfriends, they'll always rat you out.

I know right now some poor bastard is reading this saying, "Ain't that the truth."

Sorry ladies if this offends you, but it *is* the truth. Most men learn this lesson the hard way. Sometimes more than once. Take heed young dudes; women in general are not at their best when it comes to keeping secrets. Hence the saying, "Loose lips sink ships."

4. Let her vent!

As men, we tend to be problem solvers. My sister, Ginger, is fond of saying, "Men run on logic, women run on emotions." If something is broken, we have an unconscious desire to take out the old tool box and start banging things. Such is our nature. This ability serves us well when it comes to fixing the sink, or working on our car, but not so much in the emotional arena. Most of the time we don't know what we're doing anyway but our arrogance and hubris won't allow us to pull over and asks for directions.

When it comes to women, especially your woman, don't try to fix her problems. If she's upset about something that happened during her day, or a conflict with a friend, just let her vent! Do not say, "You know what I would do…" or, "Why don't you go and…." this will only provoke her more. Once again, just let her scream, yell, or cry, and keep your problem solving tool box in the garage where it belongs. Best thing you can do is put your arms around her and give her comfort and reassurance. Only if she asks for your advice, should you give it, and even then it's probably not a good idea.

5. Learn to listen.

When we communicate we do two things; we talk and listen. Some of us who are a bit loquacious tend to talk more than listen. (I guess you've surmised by now what category I belong to.) This has posed a problem for me over the years. And many a time I've heard the phrase, "You never listen to me!" To be honest, the women who blurted this out, sometimes in anger, were right. I've managed over time to learn to listen, and it's served me well. So take a deep breath, button your lips, listen to what the girl has to say, and more importantly, think before you respond. In some cases, silence is best.

6. Don't dip your pen in company ink.

Of all the places men and women meet, the workplace is more than likely number one. As tempting as it might be to start an affair with the good looking brunette from the sales department, think long and hard before going down this path. Some companies I've worked for frown on this sort of fraternization, and rightly so. The reason is obvious: If a relationship with a co-worker goes south, which is often the case, you still have to work with them. Subsequently, if you're thinking about schtupping your boss, once he or she grows tired of you, you're fired.

7. When in doubt, get out.

Why do we date? I believe we go through this process in hopes that the next person we meet will be that unique individual we can actually have a true and lasting relationship with.

Makes sense, right? Whether you know it or not, we all have a mental checklist that we employ while in the throes of that wonderful embryonic stage.

Try not to be fooled by lust. Lust is not love. In many instances you know instinctively that a new love is not right for you. But lust is a powerful aphrodisiac and you may think, "Maybe once this person realizes how special I am they'll change their ways." Not going to happen! So whether it's something as transparent as different political affiliations/religious beliefs, something as tangible as a smoking/drinking problem, or as innocuous as not putting the cap back on the toothpaste, down the road it's probably not going to work out. That is not to say you shouldn't give it a shot, everyone deserves a chance, but if there's something that just doesn't sit right with you...get out.

8. No one is as beautiful as your woman.

The next time you're sitting on the sofa with your girlfriend watching a movie starring some hot, young actress and your woman says to you, "Don't you think she's beautiful?" Turn to her, look her straight in the eye and say, "Not as beautiful as you baby." Simple.

9. Know when to take a hint.

There are very few absolutes in life but this is one of them; no matter how busy a person may be, no matter how much they have on their plate, if they want to see you, they'll make the time. The lesson is simple; if you ask someone on a date three times and they give you the runaround it means they don't want to date you. Move on.

10. The "Oouu" Factor

One of the most important components of any romantic endeavor is something I like to call the "Oouu" factor. Let's be brutally honest. (See I can be honest.) For most men, the number one factor that attracts men to women is physical beauty. It's not the only factor, but it's usually the first. And for every man, and woman for that matter, the parameters of this physical attraction vary. We all like certain types. So if you see your woman walking down the street and you don't say to yourself "Oouu, that's my woman!" all the other aspects of her being, no matter how terrific, will not carry you through.

11. Don't kiss and tell.

A true gentleman doesn't brag about his sexual encounters. There will always be one true intimate, or dear friend, that you will confide in concerning matters of the heart, but in general, the personal and private details of your sexual trysts should remain such.

12. Never marry the same woman twice.

The man who uttered this saying to me, over a half of dozen single-barrel bourbons, had a look on his face like a dog when you fake him out by pretending to throw a stick.

He went on to say, "If it didn't work the first time, why did I think it would work the second time." He then mumbled something like, "I'm such a schmuck," paid his tab, and left his words of wisdom.

13. Don't write a check with your mouth that your body can't cash.

I attribute this saying to the great, and funny, Flip Wilson. Flip is no longer with us, but is unique humor and wisdom live on. This is all part of being what we use to call in the old neighborhood, "a stand-up guy." If you make a wager with a person and you lose, pay up. If you challenge someone to a duel, (metaphorically speaking) don't back down at the last minute.

If you offer to give someone a lift to parts unknown, get a cup of coffee and be ready to roll. If you tell a woman you'll go shopping with her, don't complain when you're walking two steps behind her carrying her bags. And never tell a woman you're dynamite in bed, because if you're off your game the first time, you get the picture.

14. The Four Seasons Rule.

A very wise older gentleman imparted this insightful axiom to me many years ago. "If you're thinking about marrying someone, stay with them through four seasons before you jump the broom."

15. Posting online.

I am a computer blockhead. My last computer was so old that I bought it from Steve Jobs, out of his garage. The fact that I'm writing this on a laptop, and not some old Corona with a jar of white-out at arm's length, is a giant leap forward for me. But I know one definitive fact about this fantastical new technology: Anything you post online stays there forever for the whole world to see. That includes, friends, family, the government, and potential employers. Be careful not to hurt yourself down the road.

16. The "I love you" Dilemma.

In the throes of a new romantic adventure, passion and our old friend lust run high. Many of us are tempted to utter those three little words that change the dynamic forever. And some of us do. I think we've all been guilty of this faux pas at some time in our amorous past. There are many different kinds of love, but in the highly charged emotional arena of courtly love there are only two, "I love you because you're a wonderful person," and "I'm in love with you." I love many people, but have only been in love with a few. Use these words carefully, and make sure the other person knows which love you speak of. Above all else, don't say it unless you mean it.

17. Learn to protect yourself.

I'm not suggesting you take up Karate, albeit knowing a few good moves can come in handy. I speak of always putting yourself in a position of advantage. As you walk through life, be aware of your surroundings. Use your eyes, ears, nose and instincts, and at all times, know where you are. Whether you're riding a train, going to a nightclub, dining with friends at some new bistro, or walking on unfamiliar turf: always have an exit plan. Take a look around. Know your surroundings. Examine the people around you. Look for body language.

Let me be candid, if you find yourself in a situation where a physical confrontation might occur, qualify your position. Is the person you're dealing with drunk, high, irrational? (I'm not a tough guy, but even I smacked a drunk and knocked him down.) Are you alone or with friends? Look the person in the eye. Sometimes in instances like this a light comic remark, or a non sequitur, will defuse the situation. If you're dealing with a person who is somewhat level headed, this should be the end of it. I believe in the majority of cases like this most people really don't want to fight. Who knows, the guy might even buy you a drink. Above all else, protect yourself.

18. Never lose touch with your inner child.

Remember childhood when you found joy in the simplest things? A sheet became a tent, your room magically transformed into a racecourse or a spaceship, and toy soldiers fought the battle of Waterloo in the dirt? Your imagination was a vast canvas of new adventures as you discovered the world around you. Remember that? So what happened? This rule falls under the heading of, don't take life so seriously. No matter what your circumstance, or your station in life, learn to find joy and laughter. So the next time you break a glass, or throw your socks on the floor, and some spoilsport says, "Who did this?" Shrug your shoulders like a kid, and in your best child's voice say, "I don't know?"

19. Learn to dance

I'm not saying go out and take Rumba lessons, but a well-rounded man knows a few basic steps. This comes in handy at weddings and other such functions. Truth is, women love a man who can dance. Try this experiment: Next time you're at a wedding, or a bar mitzvah, go up to any woman and ask for a dance. I guarantee they'll say yes. Cha Cha.

20. The Spontaneity of Love

A man goes to see his psychiatrist. As they sit in his office the psychiatrist says, "So Bill, what would you like to speak about today?"

Bill replies, "Well Doc, I've been married to the same woman for fourteen years, and to be honest, the sex is kind of the same old thing."

"Well, Bill" says the doc, "my best advice to you is be more spontaneous, do it when you get the urge, catch your wife off guard, be adventurous."

The following week, Bill walks into the doctor's office and he's all smiles.

The doctor asks, "So tell me what happened?"

Bill shoots back, "Doc it was great. I was having breakfast with my wife and she dropped her fork. As she was bending down to get it, I saw part of her thigh, and I got so excited I threw everything off the table, tossed her on top of it, and schtupped her right there...it was fantastic!"

"There's just one thing though," Bill continued.

"What's that?" asked the doctor.

"We're not allowed in that restaurant anymore."

I'm not suggesting you try this, but when it comes to lovemaking, spontaneity and an adventurous spirit couldn't hurt. In the embryonic stages of a romance, being spontaneous is instinctual. For me, the first couple of go rounds with a new woman is sometimes awkward, but as time goes by, and you both start to discover each other's likes and wants, it becomes exciting and fun. As Woody Allen says, "If sex isn't disgusting, you're doing it wrong."

In today's progressive society, speaking openly about sex is acceptable behavior so don't be afraid to ask for what you want. And since none of us is a mind reader, ask your partner what turns them on. It might surprise you. If you've been with someone for a while and sex starts to feel mechanical and rote, try making love on the washing machine during the spin cycle. Take a drive in the country and do it under tree. Go to the movies and have a good old fashioned make-out session in the balcony. Or go have breakfast in a diner and get arrested for lewd and indecent behavior; use your imagination! But above all be safe, be adventurous, and have fun.

21. The First Date.

A few tips you should know about the first date:

a. Know where you're going. You can agree over the phone about where to meet, but always have a place in mind. Don't be wishy-washy. Women like confidence.

b. If you're taking her to dinner, make a reservation. If lunch, no reservation is necessary.

c. Pick her up at her door, and drop her off at her door. And (of course) open the car door for her.

d. Don't bring flowers the first time out.

e. Compliment her looks.

f. Remember rule #5. Listen to what she has to say. Let her do most of the talking.

g. Don't order food with pungent spice, like garlic or curry. Keep it light.

h. Bring an appropriate amount of cash.

i. Suggest a nightcap afterwards, or a walk in the park.

j. When you walk her to her door, as tempting as it might be, don't kiss her goodnight. If there's a connection, she'll kiss you.

22. The Bean Theorem.

At a meeting of local 348, a union rep introduces a doctor who wishes to ask a question concerning the men's sexual health. Stepping up to the microphone he says,

"How many men here are married?'

Almost all raise their hands.

"And how many of you would say you have sex with your wife a few times a week?"

A few raise their hands.

"Once a week?"

A few more raise their hands.

"Once a month?"

A spattering.

The doctor finally whittles it down to once a year. In the back of the room a lone worker frantically waves his hand. The doctor asks incredulously, "You only have sex with your wife once a year!?"

The worker excitedly replies, "That right!"

The doctor responds, "So why are you so damn happy?"

The worker says, "Tonight's the night!"

The lesson of this whimsical story is the Bean Theorem. I've heard about this experiment from many different sources with some variations but basically the same concept.

If you take a bean and put it in a jar every time you make love to a woman in the first two years of your relationship, and afterwards take a bean out every time you make love from then on, it will take you the rest of your life to empty the jar. That is not to say that after few years your lovemaking will be relegated to once a year, but it does slow down. The good thing is if it's replaced by true love and understanding, you have a shot at a real relationship. If it isn't, and your relationship is purely based on sex, you'll know it.

23. Shopping.

There are three kinds of shopping: The man way, the woman way, and window shopping. Men shop very differently than women do. For most women shopping is an adventure, for most men it's a chore. Men go to the store for a predetermined item: we walk in, buy it and walk out. This is the way we do business with most of the everyday stuff we purchase. We don't shop, we buy. That's what we were built to do. In and out. And during the occasional moments we do go browsing, it's usually in the tool department of Home Depot which is as alien to women as the lingerie department in Macy's is to us.

So what's the rule here? If your woman wants to go for a stroll through the mall to window shop, have some lunch, and go see a movie, by all means—have fun. But if the lady in question is in "Shopping Mode," my best advice is to steer clear. Dragging yourself two paces behind a woman on the seemingly endless mission to find that "perfect pair of pumps" is tantamount to being stuck in an airport for several hours with nothing to read, nothing to drink, and no one to converse with.

So the next time your woman says, "Honey I'm going shopping, would you like to come?" be honest. If you want to, great. If not, say, "No, that's okay, have fun." You'll thank me for it.

24. Don't tell her everything.

I once dated a free spirited woman who told me that it didn't bother her to hear of my amorous adventures as a young musician, gallivanting through life schtupping everything that moved. So... being the immature, garrulous blabbermouth that I was, I constantly regaled her with stories of my exploits knocking around New York City with my motley crew of equally debaucherous and depraved young dudes.

If I ran into an old girlfriend, I made absolutely no effort to hide the extent of my relationship from the woman in question. I thought to myself, "This is great. I finally met a woman who doesn't care how many other chicks I've been with!" (This is the true definition of the word, "Schmuck") One evening, while walking to a movie theatre on 59th St., I mentioned that the last time I was at this particular location I was dating some chick from NYU.

The woman blew-up in my face! She screamed that she was sick and tired of hearing my tales of sex, drugs and rock n' roll, and if I didn't cease and desist she would break my nose, cut off my testicles, and burn my guitar! Wow! But that dear reader is not the moral of this story.

I continued to see this person, and every time we had a disagreement or lover's spat, she brought up my sordid past. Every party we attended was followed by a slew of questions concerning some woman who paid too much attention to me, or I to her.

The truth is: no matter how open minded someone may seem, I believe no one wants to hear about your affairs before you met them, and I was a fool to fall into that trap. (I told you I was a schmuck.) Mind you, none of us are monks and most will know that you had a life, and loves, before you met them, but *knowing* that fact is totally different than being constantly reminded of it.

This rule falls under the heading of, "what she doesn't know won't hurt her." That is not to say I'm advocating having an affair or lying, but when speaking of your other life before you met your soulmate, learn to couch your words carefully. I've gone from, "I went to the Met with Jane" to "I saw a concert here with a friend." And most importantly, the next time a woman questions you about your sordid days and says, "Come on, tell me, I won't get angry," don't.

25. Create your own style.

Whether it's a pencil moustache, a retro haircut, a carnation in your lapel, an ascot, or distinctive eyewear, create something that's uniquely you. I don a sports jacket almost every day. I feel comfortable in it, and it's become a part of who I am. Try to find that one thing that sets you apart from the crowd.

26. Cats and Dogs

Knowing how sensitive people are about this subject, I'd like to preface this essay by stating emphatically that I don't dislike pets. When it comes to the domestic varieties, cats and dogs, I'm a dog person. Unless your pet is a wolverine or a jackal, there are no bad pets, just bad pet owners.

Dogs and cats are like children who never grow up. And like children, the one thing they need most in their lives is consistency. If you're a married man with a house, children, and big backyard, having a loyal canine is a welcome addition to family life. Dogs are very communal, love people, are protective, and in my opinion, the best alarm system you can have. You'll never hear a burglar say, "Frankie, they got cats!" If a dog is fed at the same time every day, walked at the same time, and let out in the backyard to play every day, everybody's happy. Once this pattern is broken, or if it never existed to begin with, it's almost assured that you'll have problems with a pet.

The fault lies not with "Scruffy," but with his owner. It's not the dog's fault it pooped on the rug, it's your fault. If you're a single guy who goes out all the time, has a few drinks with friends after work, and plays in a rock band, my advice is simple; don't own a dog! Because ultimately all the bad things that happen in your apartment while you're gone, from poop on the floor, a garbage pail turned over, your dog destroying your CD collection, and curtains being ripped off the windows, to disturbing your neighbors who are now pissed at you...is your fault, not the dog's.

A dog or cat is not a toy that you can throw away when you grow tired of it. This is one of the reasons there are so many strays. According to the Humane Society, from 2012-2013, 2.7 million dogs and cats were euthanized in the United States alone. If you do decide to own a pet, get it neutered, and make sure your lifestyle is compatible for pet ownership. Also, research the breed. Depending on how you live, make sure the breed of dog fits. You don't want a dog who's too big for your place, too aggressive, chews your furniture, sheds a great deal, etc. Do your homework.

Now granted, cats are much easier to care for, but if you're someone who moves around, not every rental will accept pets and some want a $10-$20 a month fee for each animal you own. But owning a pet isn't cheap: feeding, grooming, licensing, the occasional trip to the vet and any other cost your particular pet might incur. You should consider all these factors before owning a pet. I could go on *ad infinitum* concerning my personal trials and adventures with the animal kingdom, but that would be voluminous. Instead, I will leave you with a quote from a famous TV character, "Fish make good pets...you don't have to walk them or pet them, and by the time you get sick of them...they die." Thank you Archie Bunker.

27. Be a Man.

This might sound like an antiquated notion, but for all the bad things that man has done over the centuries, we've also achieved great heights. Every magical cathedral or fantastic skyscraper you've ever seen or been in, was built by men. Men sailed in wooden ships and discovered the world. All the art that adorns the museums of the Renaissance was created by men. Every renowned classical composer was a man. Men dug the Panama Canal. Men landed on the moon.

None of these achievements are meant to diminish women's contributions to world. Women were the inspiration for most, if not all, of these accomplishments. And atrocities such as the wars and the killing that men have perpetrated on society, albeit immeasurable, should not diminish the impact of man's contribution to society. I believe the influence and inspiration of women has tempered our modern culture, and we're better off for it. But as men, we should be proud of our place in the world. So hold your head high.

When you walk into a place, act like you own it. Carry yourself with purpose. Exude confidence. Be a man of your own convictions. Say what you mean and mean what you say. Try to always look your best, you never know who you'll run into. Never act arrogant or haughty. Do good deeds. Look people in the eye. Avoid gossip. Always try to take the high road. Tell your family and friends you love and appreciate them.

Take care of those you love. After all is said and done, remember the line from H.G. Wells *The Island of Dr. Moreau*, "Are we not men?"

7

The Grasshopper and the Ant

A few weeks ago, I celebrated my sixtieth birthday. Not really a great accomplishment, although I wonder sometimes how I made it this far, considering the peripatetic gypsy-esque life I've led.

Some events in this colorful journey I had no control over, but for the most part, this is the life I chose. Unlike most, unable to decide what they wanted to be when they grew up, I at a very tender age knew exactly what I wanted my course to be. I wanted to be in Show-Biz. So, after a thirty year odyssey of playing music, and another ten years of acting, stand-up, directing and playwriting, I find myself here, where it all began: writing.

I look back and question my decisions. Did I say, "No" when I should have said, "Yes?" Did I zig when I should have zagged? All artists do this. In the end, there is no correct answer. I know I am not alone in this. The history books are filled with artists, brilliant or otherwise, who in the end die penniless and alone. And for every famous actor or singer you see on TV whose career is going well, there are thousands of others passing out their headshots, waiting for the phone to ring. So what is it that drives the creative mind to live a life that in most cases is inimical to one's well-being? I refer to this as, "The Grasshopper Life." Allow me to explain. Most of us know the parable of the grasshopper and the ant. For those who don't, here is the version I know:

Deep in the woods among the vast expanse of the forest floor lived an ant and a grasshopper. Mr. Ant and his family resided in a hollowed out knot at the base of a mighty oak tree. Spring had just blossomed as the trees and foliage burst to life in bucolic splendor. With only a short reprise to enjoy the beauty of spring, and the warmth of summer, the ant and his family immediately went to work gathering fruits and nuts for the following winter.

Across the grassy plain, in a weathered patch of grass, lived the grasshopper. Awakening from his slumber, the grasshopper went right to work doing what he did best: playing music, painting, singing, dancing, and totally enjoying the company of his friends, seemingly without a care in the world. All the while the frugal, industrious ant toiled away making sure he and his family would have enough when the cold winter winds blew again.

As the weeks passed, one day the ant, curious of the grasshopper, made his way across the grassy meadow and approached the grasshopper's flimsy abode. The grasshopper, pencil in hand, was sketching a female grasshopper. The ant broke the silence, "Mr. Grasshopper might I have a word with you?"

"What can I do for you Mr. Ant?"

"Well…" said the ant, "Mr. Grasshopper, I know it's none of my business how you live your life, but as the summer draws to a close, I've noticed that you've gathered no provisions for the winter. How do you intend to survive?"

The grasshopper perked up, "Well, I'm having a big opening in a gallery downtown next week. And I am very close to selling a screenplay that I wrote. And then there's a record company that seems very interested in my music, so as soon as one of those deals breaks, I should be in the chips!"

The ant took a deep breath and said, "And what if none of those things happen Mr. Grasshopper, what will you do then?"

"Do you doubt my talent Mr. Ant?" replied the Grasshopper.

"Not at all," said Mr. Ant. "But having talent, and making a living at it, are two totally different things." He continued, "What I'm trying to say is, what will you eat, where will you sleep, when the winter comes?"

The grasshopper paused and thought for a moment, "I try my best not to think about such things. I know in my heart that one day I'll be rich and famous, move out of this forest, and live in the big city!" The grasshopper turned back to his female model and said, "Now, if you'll pardon me Mr. Ant, I must get back to my life's work."

"Good day Mr. Grasshopper," said the ant.

"Good day Mr. Ant," said the grasshopper.

As the ant made his way back to his humble abode, he turned to see some of the grasshopper's friends pulling up on motorcycles. Carrying cases of beer and bottles of Jack Daniels, they launched a party that would last more than a week, and this enthusiastic, creative, and sometimes frivolous behavior would continue through the rest of the season. All the while, the assiduous ant, and his assiduous ant family, gathered provisions for the long cold winter ahead.

One night, as frost lay upon the deciduous remains of the forest, the ant sitting by his fireside reading a newspaper, heard a knock at his door. Getting up, he called out, "Who is it that knocks at my door this late hour?"

"It is I, the grasshopper!"

The ant cracked the door a notch, "What do you want Mr. Grasshopper?"

"May I come in Mr. Ant?" said the grasshopper.

"No you may not!" the ant replied.

The grasshopper buried his head in his shoulders against the bitter wind as the ant continued, "What do you want Mr. Grasshopper?"

"I am cold and hungry Mr. Ant, and in dire need of shelter from the storm. Won't you please help me?"

"Why should I help you?!" the ant barked.

"Because I'm your neighbor" chattered the grasshopper

"What happened to all your grandiose plans?" asked the ant.

The grasshopper replied in slow, measured tones that reflected his defeat, "Things just didn't work out the way I thought they would. My record deal fell through, my art didn't sell, and my screenplay was turned down. You see, Mr. Ant, it's just a minor setback. I'll be good as new come next spring. If you could just put me up for a little while, I promise I'll be no bother."

The ant looked sternly at the grasshopper and said, "I am sorry Mr. Grasshopper, but I cannot help you. Maybe if you had taken my advice, you wouldn't be in this mess."

With that, the ant closed the door and bolted it shut. The grasshopper fought his way back to his wind-blown lean-to. As he covered himself with some leaves from an art book and an old Yardbirds album, he cursed his fate and shivered himself to sleep. By the time the winter sun broke through the trees, and the sound of the mourning birds breached the silence of the dawn, the grasshopper was dead.

Boo, Hoo, Hoo.

So, as they say, what's the moral of this melancholy tale? For anyone who managed to graduate the sixth grade, and has a modicum of intelligence, the initial inference is clear. Our lexicon of quotations is filled with such staunch reminders as, "A penny saved is a penny earned." "Don't count your chickens before they hatch." "A bird in the hand is worth two in the bush." "A fool and his money are soon parted." And so on.

All valuable life lessons that regale the virtues of hard work, frugality, perseverance and saving for a rainy day. And since I'm guessing that the life-cycles of insects are miniscule in comparison to other more advanced life forms, the analogies are obvious. The summer represents youth: the winter, old age. But was the grasshopper any less stalwart in his pursuit of his dream? Or were his aspirations too lofty and intangible, as dreams often are? Allow me to present an alternative ending to this story.

As autumn turned to winter, the ant saw very little of his grasshopper neighbor. He continued to stockpile supplies and proceeded to hunker down for the long winter months ahead. As the frost eventually melted away, and the first signs of spring filled the air, the ant was awakened to the sound of heavy equipment rumbling passed his tree trunk abode. Peering out his window, he saw a bulldozer knocking down the remains of the grasshopper's shack as a small team of hard hats surveyed the area. He thought to himself, "Good riddance!"

In the next few weeks, a vast construction site arose around the grasshopper's old habitat. Eventually, a beautiful home graced the site of the old run-down lean-to. The ant was upbeat, "Maybe this time I'll get a decent neighbor instead of that good-for-nothing grasshopper."

One day while tending his garden with some of his ant children, a flashy sports car with the top down pulled up in front of the ant's property. Much to the surprise and dismay of the ant, it was the grasshopper. Beside him sat a very thin, stunning, young female. The grasshopper greeted the ant exuberantly, "Hello Mr. Ant, so nice to see you again!"

The ant replied callously, "I wish I could say the same."

"Oh come now, don't be that way" said the grasshopper. "After all, we're soon to be

neighbors again!"

The ant was incredulous. "You mean to say that house across the way is yours?"

The grasshopper continued happily, "Well, actually it's my summer home."

The ant stood in bewildered silence as the grasshopper went on, "You see Mr. Ant, I've had a string of good luck lately. It seems that after my opening in the city, I got a rave review from the *New York Times*, and my solo album just went platinum, which prompted the sale of my screenplay, which is being made into a movie as we speak!" As a side note, he proclaimed, "I think I'll have Spielberg direct it!"

With that the grasshopper said, "Peace out my brother," put the car in gear, and sped away across the forest floor. The ant stood flustered. All summer long he was an irate witness to the never-ending parties and Rock n' Roll debauchery emanating from the summer home of the now famous and revered talk of the town. The grasshopper magnanimously invited the ant, and his family, to every outing, but the stoic ant never showed.

Now I know this second scenario doesn't happen much, and the odds are great against it, but it does happen! More important is the question: what is it that makes some if us grasshoppers and some of us ants? Knowing the odds are greater than winning the sweepstakes, why does the grasshopper persist? For some it is the allure of money, others the fame. But for the truly talented, the answer is simple: he or she has something to say, something undeniably important that the world needs to know, or so they believe.

Grasshoppers have an inexorable need to leave their mark on society. The monies that might be made from their ventures (albeit a beneficial side effect) in most cases are not the main objective. Currently, our cultural society is saturated with untalented hacks, some famous just for being famous, who make tons of money, but will be lucky if they're a footnote in the annals of history. (It is worth noting that Van Gogh sold only one painting during his lifetime, and even more drastic than his infamous act of cutting his ear off, was shooting himself in the chest at the age of thirty-seven, broke and alone.) This enduring desire to be heard is what drives the true grasshopper spirit. To some it is a blessing, to most a curse.

What is to be learned by this parable of these two dichotomous insects? What would the world be like if only one of these ideologies existed? Let's first examine the ant. We're all aware of the virtues of self-reliance and hard work. It's this form of tenacious and indefatigable drive that built our civilization. But as they say, "all work and no play makes Jack a dull boy." In other words, the world at large would be a pretty dull place if all its inhabitants were ants. That is in no way meant to diminish the great accomplishments of individual and collective hard labor, for the ant's contribution to mankind is indisputable and indispensable. This bedrock commitment for the betterment of society can be seen all around us, every day.

On the altruistic side, we have the grasshopper. Head in the clouds, dreaming of utopia, his contributions can also be seen, heard and read. He aspires to feed the soul; to ennoble the mind; to write the history of mankind's poetic journeys; to create the sounds and sensations of the human spirit. But if only his view of life existed it might resemble Gulliver's travels to the land of Laputa where alchemic and ethereal pursuits produce nothing of practical use.

So what to do if you're a grasshopper? Know that the grasshopper's life is usually filled with many disappointments. There is no set formula to success in his world, and those who are driven by one purpose either exceed in their dreams or fall from a great height. That is not to say don't try, but as they say in show-biz, "Don't quit your day job just yet."

The ancient Greeks were fond of saying, "all things in moderation." This is wise advice. There's always a middle ground. Through many years of playing music, writing, acting, and doing stand-up, I've always had a job. I wish I could say I've made a living from loftier pursuits, but that would be untrue. I had fun like our friend the grasshopper and to this day continue to pursue my dreams. So my advice: if you're a musician, actor, dancer, painter, or a poet, try to be both an Ant and a Grasshopper. Find a line of employment you can tolerate and pursue your dream on the side. In the end, you never know, you just might get lucky, and if not, at least you'll have some great and colorful stories to tell the kiddies.

Peace out, fellow Grasshoppers!

Acknowledgments

I would first like to acknowledge the one person that's truly responsible for this small self-help guide to grooming and beyond reaching fruition. Dr. Patricia Ross, Senior Editor at Hugo House Publishing, has been nothing short of a guide, mentor, soundboard, psychiatrist, babysitter and hopefully, I'd like to think, a friend. (She assures me, it's true). She has walked me through every step of this process, never once losing her temper or becoming short with me even when I questioned her knowledge of the comma. (What was I thinking? There isn't a "Doctor" before her name for nothing!) In short this book wouldn't exist without her. Thanks Doc.

Which leads me to her colleague, Christa Mella, whose dedication and unwavering professionalism has given this book life.

To Eric Cooper, my son, who helped with my never ending tech questions and woes and designed the periodic images that appear on the pages.

And finally Paula Sinnard, to whom this book is dedicated. Stunning and graceful. Always looking sharp with a keen sense of fashion and style. She's one of those amazing women who could wear sackcloth and make it look good.

About the Author

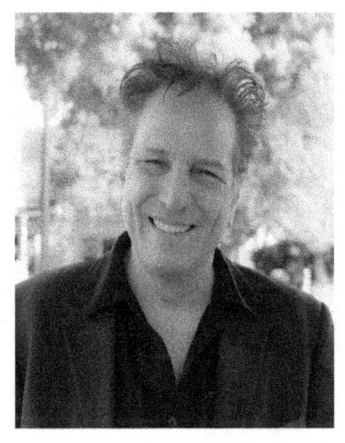

Sal Cipolla is a produced playwright, an award-winning film director who has appeared in many short- and feature-length films. He is also a musician, an actor, a stand-up comic and most of all a raconteur. He currently resides in Austin, TX.

If you would like to comment or leave a note for the author.Please write to mrsalexcellentguide@gmail.com.

www.ingramcontent.com/pod-product-compliance
Lightning Source LLC
Chambersburg PA
CBHW070450050426
42451CB00015B/3427